NEUROSURGERY ORAL BOARD REVIEW

André des Etages

Thieme

NEUROSURGERY ORAL BOARD REVIEW

Jonathan Stuart Citow, M.D.
Chairman
Division of Neurosurgery
Condell Medical Center
Libertyville, Illinois
and
Clinical Assisstant Professor
Section of Neurosurgery
University of Chicago Medical Center
Chicago, Illinois

Coauthor and Illustrator
Lydia M. Johns
University of Chicago Medical Center
Chicago, Illinois

Thieme

New York · Stuttgart

Thieme Medical Publishers, Inc.
333 Seventh Ave.
New York, NY 10001

Editor: Felicity Edge
Editorial Assistant: Jennifer Berger
Director, Production and Manufacturing: Anne Vinnicombe
Production Editor: Becky Dille
Marketing Director: Phyllis Gold
Sales Manager: Ross Lumpkin
Chief Financial Officer: Peter van Woerden
President: Brian D. Scanlan
Compositor: Thomson Press International
Printer: Maple-Vail Book Manufacturing Group

Library of Congress Cataloging-in-Publication Data

Citow, Jonathan Stuart.
Neurosurgery oral board review / Jonathan Stuart Citow ; co-author and illustrator, Lydia M. Johns.
p. ; cm.
ISBN 1-58890-162-9 (TMP : alk. paper) -- ISBN 3-13-135771-1 (GTV : alk. paper)
1. Nervous sytem--Surgery--Examinations, questions, etc. I. Johns, Lydia M. II. Title.
[DNLM; 1. Neurosurgical Procedures--Examination Questions. WL 18.2 C581n 2003]
RD593.C488 2003
317
4′8′0076--dc21 2002042995

Important note: Medical knowledge is ever-changing. As new research and clinical experience broaden our knowledge, changes in treatment and drug therapy may be required. The authors and editors of the material herein have consulted sources believed to be reliable in their efforts to provide information that is complete and in accord with the standards accepted at the time of publication. However, in the view of the possibility of human error by the authors, editors, or publisher, of the work herein, or changes in medical knowledge, neither the authors, editors, or publisher, nor any other party who has been involved in the preparation of this work, warrants that the information contained herein is in every respect accurate or complete, and they are not responsible for any errors or omissions or for the results obtained from use of such information. Readers are encouraged to confirm the information contained herein with other sources. For example, readers are advised to check the product information sheet included in the package of each drug they plan to administer to be certain that the information contained in this publication is accurate and that changes have not been made in the recommended dose or in the contraindications for administration. This recommendation is of particular importance in connection with new or infrequently used drugs. Some of the product names, patents, and registered designs referred to in this book are in fact registered trademarks or proprietary names even though specific reference to this fact is not always made in the text. Therefore, the appearance of a name without designation as proprietary is not to be construed as a representation by the publisher that it is in the public domain.

Printed in the United States of America

5 4 3 2 1

TMP ISBN 1-58890-162-9
GTV ISBN 3 13 135771 1

Dedication

This book is dedicated to my wife Karen who has graciously run our household and managed my life while I have toiled on this one last book (I promise). It is also dedicated to my children Benjamin and Emma who have only accidentally unplugged the computer seven times while I have been typing this manuscript. I am beginning to suspect that it was intentional. Okay, now we can go skating . . .

CONTENTS

PREFACE

I wrote this book using the notes that I scribbled down while studying for the neurosurgery oral board examination. This book is not intended to serve as a replacement for the classic neurosurgical texts, but as a supplement to the knowledge gained during the long years of residency and in the early stages of practice. I tried to focus on the major aspects of diseases that a neurosurgeon may encounter, both in clinical practice and on the examination. For a more thorough helping of knowledge, consider thumbing through the texts in the reference list. My favorite is *Comprehensive Neurosurgical Board Review*, but I may be a little biased. That book was geared for the written boards, but the anatomy, pathology/radiology, neurology, and neurosurgery sections provide useful information that is not covered in this text.

I must admit that I was a tad intimidated by the oral examination before I lived through it. I expected to hear "So, Dr. Citow, can you please show me the incision for the hypoglossal-pundendal nerve anastomsas used for people who constantly speak out of their asses." But it really was a fair test and a surprisingly pleasant experience. I truly got the sense that the examiners are out to reinforce their preconceived notion that the examinee (you) is indeed competent (not the other way around) and makes reasonable decisions. They are not out to trick you with obscure details. Stay relaxed and suggest exactly what you would do in everyday practice (not in a surreal ivory tower university setting) and all will be fine. The only disheartening aspect of the test is that none of the examiners smile (but this may be their baseline state) or acknowledge that you are correct (but neither do your patients in the hospital, unless they have been on the Internet. . . .) Good luck!

INTRODUCTION

Relax, there is little they will ask you that you have not treated successfully numerous times. Remember, this book is one person's view of things. There are many ways to skin a nerve root. As long as the patients are well cared for, all will be fine

REFERENCES

Neurological Surgery, 4th Edition. Youmans JR (Ed.). Philadelphia, PA:W.B. Saunders, Inc., 1994.

Handbook of Neurosurgery, 5th Edition. Greenberg MS. New York, NY: Thieme Medical Publishers, 2001.

Principles of Neurology, 5th Edition. Adams RD, Victor M. New York, NY:McGraw Hill, 1993.

Comprehensive Neurosurgical Board Review. Citow JS. New York, NY: Thieme Medical Publishers, 2000

The following journals provided information:

Journal of Neurosurgery

Neurosurgery

Surgical Neurology

CHAPTER 1

ANATOMY

I. PTERION

A. Junction of frontal, parietal, temporal, and greater wing of sphenoid bones

B. Located two fingerbreadths above the zygomatic arch and two finger widths behind the frontal process of zygoma (Fig. 1–1)

II. ASTERION

A. Junction of lambdoid, parietomastoid, and occipitomastoid sutures

B. Located over the transverse–sigmoid junction.

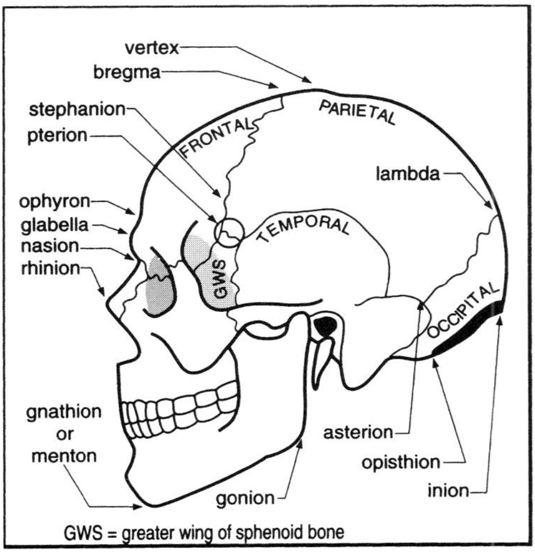

Figure 1–1 Craniometric points. (With permission from Greenberg MS. Handbook of Neurosurgery. *5th ed. New York, NY: Thieme Medical Publishers; 2001:96, Fig. 3–2.)*

III. Bregma

A. Junction of coronal–sagittal suture

IV. Frankfort Plane

A. From inferior orbit to top of external acoustic meatus (EAM)

V. Posterior Ear Line

A. Midmastoid up rostrally perpendicular to baseline (Frankfort plane)

VI. Sylvian Fissure

A. Lateral canthus to $\frac{3}{4}$ of nasion–inion line and ending at posterior ear line.

VII. Motor Strip

A. Four to 5 cm behind coronal suture; top is at posterior ear line and direction is 45 degrees from Frankfort baseline

VIII. Central Sulcus

A. Top is 2 cm behind $\frac{2}{4}$ nasion–inion line (3–4 cm behind coronal suture); bottom is 5 cm above EAM

IX. Angular Gyrus

A. Located just above the pinna; caps the superior temporal sulcus

B. Wernicke's receptive speech area also includes the supramarginal gyrus that caps the sylvian fissure.

X. Broca's Area

A. Expressive speech center located in inferior frontal gyrus pars opercularis (behind the pars orbitalis and triangularis)

XI. Superior Orbital Fissure Contents

A. Cranial nerves III, IV, V1 (all three branches: nasociliary, frontal, and lacrimal), VI

B. Sympathetic fibers from the ICA plexus

C. Superior orbital vein

D. Orbital branch of the middle meningeal artery

E. Recurrent meningeal branch of the lacrimal artery.

XII. Inferior Orbital Fissure

A. Cranial nerve V2

B. Zygomatic nerve

C. Pterygopalatine branch of the maxillary nerve

D. Infraorbital artery and vein

E. Inferior ophthalmic vein

XIII. Orbital Tendinous Ring (Annulus of Zinn)

A. Structures passing above it include the lacrimal nerve, the frontal nerve, and cranial nerve IV.

B. Structures passing through it include the superior and inferior divisions of cranial nerve III, the nasociliary nerve, and cranial nerve VI.

C. Mnemonic device—*l*uscious (lacrimal) *F*rench (frontal) *t*arts (trochlear) / *s*tand (superior division III) *n*aked (nasociliary) *i*n (inferior division III) *a*nticipation (abducens) (Fig. 1–2)

XIV. Circle of Willis

A. Complete in only 20% of the population

XV. Fetal Circulation

A. ICA supplies the posterior circulation (occurs in 25% of the population)

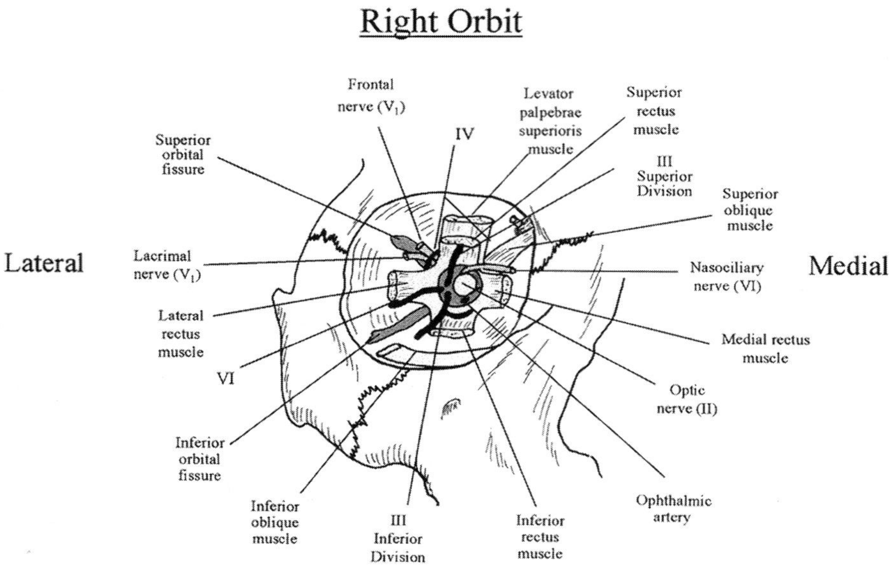

Figure 1–2 *Tendinous ring. (With permission from Citow JS.* Comprehensive Neurosurgical Board Review. *New York, NY: Thieme Medical Publishers; 2000:76, Fig. 1–41.)*

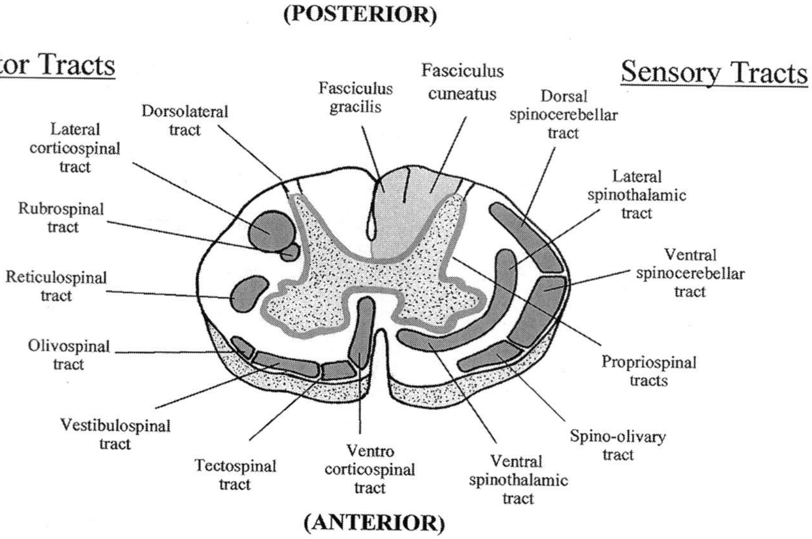

Figure 1–3 *Spinal cord pathways. (With permission from Citow JS.* Comprehensive Neurosurgical Board Review. *New York, NY: Thieme Medical Publishers; 2000:69, Fig. 1–39.)*

XVI. Vertebral Artery

A. Enters the foramen transversarium at C6

B. Distal to the C1 foramina transversarium, it curves posteromedially toward the lamina of C1 and then pierces the dura to move anterosuperomedially toward the anterior brain stem.

XVII. Artery of Adamkiewicz

A. Usually enters the spinal canal on the left at T9–12 to supply T8 to the conus

XVIII. Spinal Tracts

A. Upper extremities are medial in the corticospinal tracts and spinothalamic tracts.

B. Lower extremities are medial in the posterior columns (Figs. 1–3 and 1–4).

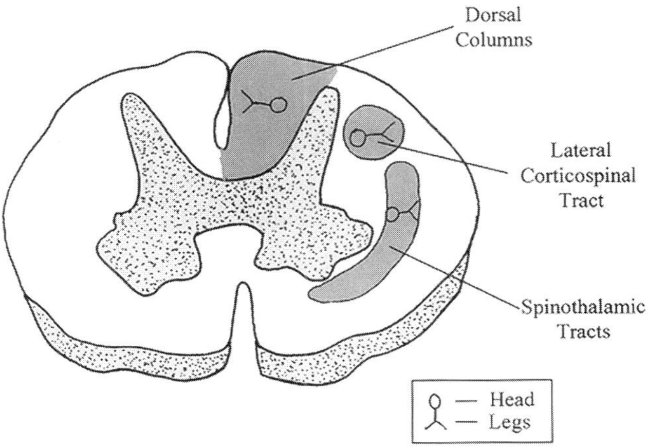

Figure 1–4 Spinal cord somatotopic organization. (With permission from Citow JS. Comprehensive Neurosurgical Board Review. *New York, NY: Thieme Medical Publishers; 2000:70, Fig. 1–40.)*

CHAPTER 2

Critical Care and Neuroanesthesia

I. Shock

A. Hypovolemic—there is usually a 30% decrease in blood volume before there is impaired organ perfusion.

B. Cardiogenic—due to impaired cardiac pumping

C. Septic—due to lowered peripheral vascular resistance, usually associated with gram-negative rods

D. Neurogenic—due to decreased sympathetic output causing lowered peripheral vascular resistance, with blood pooling in veins after a spinal cord injury

II. Adrenal Insufficiency

A. Low adrenocorticotropic hormone (ACTH)—can usually be replaced with just glucocorticoid (dexamethasone)

B. Primary adrenal insufficiency (Addison's disease)—must be treated with mineral and glucocorticoids (hydrocortisone or prednisone). Patients on steroids for > 2 weeks must be tapered off over 2 weeks.

C. Symptomatic adrenal insufficiency—includes fatigue, hypotension, hypoglycemia, hyponatremia, hyperkalemia, and hyperthermia

III. Hypothyroidism

A. Signs/Symptoms—usually fatigue, coarse hair, cold intolerance, constipation, and possibly neurological impairment

B. Myxedema coma—includes hypotension, bradycardia, hypothermia, hyponatremia, and hypoglycemia with a 50% mortality. T_3 is the active form of the hormone.

IV. Syndrome of Inappropriate Antidiuretic Hormone (SIADH)

A. Normovolemia—serum osmolarity < 280, urine osmolarity $>$ serum osm, serum $Na^+ < 135$ mEq/L, and urine $Na^+ > 50$ mEq/L

B. Urine output—usually low (~40–60 mL/h)

C. Urine Na^+—usually close to 50 mEq/L

D. Treatment—fluid restriction 1 L/d, NaCl 3% 30 mL IV q1h × 3 and Lasix to reach 125 to 130 mEq/L. Avoid rapid correction more than 1 mEq/L/h to avoid central pontine myelinolysis. Consider adding demeclocycline 300 mg PO q8h or lithium 300 mg PO q8h to cause nephrogenic diabetes insipidus in refractory cases.

V. Cerebral Salt Wasting

A. Hypovolemia—with loss of free water and Na^+

B. Decreased weight and central venous pressure (CVP)

C. Urine output—usually high ($>$ 100 mL/h)

D. Urine Na^+—usually around 130 mEq/L

E. Treatment—0.9% normal saline boluses

VI. Diabetes Insipidus

A. Urine output—$>$ 300 mL/h × 3, specific gravity < 1.005

B. Urine Na^+—$<$ 10 mEq/L, serum $Na^+ > 145$. Watch to differentiate from normal postoperative diuresis that maintains a normal serum Na^+.

C. Treatment—fluid replacement of $\frac{1}{2}$ normal saline (NS) and desmopressin acetate (DDAVP) 0.1 to 0.2 μg IV q8h. Long-term care may require intranasal DDAVP 10 to 40 μg b.i.d.

VII. Transfusion Reactions

A. Hemolytic—caused by ABO blood incompatability

1. Signs/Symptoms—lumbar pain, disseminated intravascular coagulopathy (DIC), and shock
2. Treatment—stop the transfusion and diurese with mannitol and fluids

B. Allergic—caused by antibodies to plasma proteins

1. Signs/Symptoms—hives
2. Treatment—Benadryl. The transfusion usually does not need to be stopped.

C. Febrile—caused by antibodies to donor white blood cells (WBCs)

1. Signs/Symptoms—fever
2. Treatment—Tylenol. The transfusion usually does not need to be stopped. Send off blood for analysis to rule out hemolysis.

VIII. Anaphylaxis

1. Treatment—epinephrine 1:1000 0.5 mL SQ, Benadryl 50 mg IM, and Decadron 10 mg IV

IX. Deep Vein Thrombosis

1. Prevent with TED hose, sequential compression devices, and heparin SQ 5000 mg b.i.d. or Lovenox 30 mg SQ b.i.d.
2. Rule out pulmonary embolus with ventilation–perfusion (V/Q) scan, spiral CT, or pulmonary angiogram.
3. Treatment—anticoagulation or Greenfield inferior vena cava filter

X. Coumadin

A. Weaning off for surgery

1. Patients with a mechanical heart valve—stop the Coumadin for 2 days then admit to the hospital for heparin

2. Patients with atrial fibrillation—stop the Coumadin 5 days before surgery. It is usually safe to resume heparin 5 days after a craniotomy.

XI. Pre-Op Analgesia

A. Decadron 10 mg IV, Torodol 30 mg IV, and Marcaine 0.5% SQ and IM.

XII. Preintubation Treatment

A. Denitrogenation with 100% O_2 for 5 minutes. Atropine to decrease the vagal cardiac response and secretions. Lidocaine 100 mg IV to decrease pharyngeal reactivity and intracranial pressure (ICP)

XIII. Competitive Muscle Blockade

A. Reverse from pancuronium with neostigmine and atropine or glycopyrrolate.

XIV. Evoked Potential Monitoring

A. Avoid inhalation agents; nitrous oxide and narcotics preferred. Short-acting muscle relaxants are okay, but not benzodiazepines or barbiturates.

B. Turn off nitrous oxide 10 minutes before dural closure to avoid tension pneumocephalus.

XV. Malignant Hyperthermia

A. Hypermetabolic state of skeletal muscle due to an idiopathic block of calcium reentry into the sarcoplasmic reticulum causing increased oxygen consumption

B. Fifty percent of patients have had normal anesthesia.

C. Increased incidence with halothane and succinylcholine

D. Temperature may increase to 44°C (113°F) at 1° per 5 minutes.

E. Watch for increased pCO_2, decreased pO_2, tachycardia, DIC, acidosis, rigid limbs, increased creatine phosphokinase (CPK), and ultimately hypotension and death.

F. Patients are normally hypothermic with anesthesia.

G. Treatment—stop the anesthesia; change the tubing; administer dantrolene sodium and 100% O_2; lower the core temperature with cool IV fluids; perform wound, nasogastric, and rectal irrigation; administer bicarbonate to decrease acidosis, and insulin and glucose to decrease K^+.

H. Test preoperatively with a muscle biopsy to see if it contracts to halothane or caffeine.

I. Watch for masseter spasm after injection of succinylcholine during the case.

CHAPTER 3

NEUROLOGY

I. DEMENTIA

A. Treatable causes (20%)—medications, alcohol (ETOH), heavy metals, central nervous system (CNS) infection, hyperthyroidism, hypothyroidism, hyperglycemia, hypoglycemia, decreased parathyroid hormone (PTH), hypopituitarism, hyponatremia, Cushing's disease, Wilson's disease, uremia, porphyria, hydrochephalus, chronic subdural hematoma, tumor, hypertension, deficiency of vitamin B_1, B_{12}, or folate

B. Untreatable causes (80%)—Alzheimer's disease (50%), multi-infarct dementia (15%), Pick's disease, progressive supranuclear palsy (PSNP, Steele-Richardson-Olszewski syndrome), Parkinson's disease, Huntington's chorea, multiple sclerosis (MS), systemic lupus erythematosis (SLE), sarcoid, progressive multifocal leukoencephalopathy (PML), and Creutzfeldt-Jakob disease (CJD).

C. Evaluation—CBC (infection or B_{12}/folate deficiency with MCV >100); electrolytes (glucose, Na^+, BUN); thyroid; B_{12}; folate; urine toxicity screen; electrocardiogram (EKG) (AFib with lacunes); chest x-ray (CXR), computed tomography (CT), lumbar puncture (LP), Venereal Disease Research Laboratory (VDRL).

II. WERNICKE'S ENCEPHALOPATHY

A. Cause—thiamin deficiency, usually in alcoholics

B. Signs/Symptoms—confusion, conjugate gaze and lateral rectus palsies, nystagmus, and gait ataxia

C. Evaluation—MRI may detect inflammation and necrosis of the mamillary bodies, periventricular thalamus and hypothalamus, periaqueductal gray, floor of the fourth ventricle, and superior cerebellar vermis.

D. Treatment—thiamin 100 mg IV followed by daily supplements and a normal diet

E. Korsakoff's psychosis—a more chronic disorder with short-term memory loss and learning difficulties

III. Creutzfeldt-Jakob Disease

A. Cause—prion or slow virus

B. Signs/Symptoms—dementia, ataxia, visual loss, and myoclonus

C. Evaluation—MRI (hyperintense on T2 in basal ganglia), LP (rule out syphilis, may see increased protein), EEG (periodic spikes), and biopsy (spongiform encephalitis with decreased cells and no inflammation, stain for protease-resistent protein).

D. Treatment—no treatment, death usually within 1 year

E. Precaution—sterilize biopsy equipment with steam and sodium hydroxide.

IV. Progressive Supranuclear Palsy (PSNP, Steele-Richardson-Olszewski Syndrome)

A. Cause—unknown, possibly autoimmune

B. Signs/Symptoms—progressive deterioration in intellect, speech, vision, gait, voluntary eye control, and pseudobulbar palsy. Most patients are 50 to 60 years old and male.

C. Evaluation—mainly clinical. MRI may show atrophy of the midbrain, superior colliculus, and subthalamic nuclei.

D. Treatment—none

V. Parkinsonism

A. Cause—substantia nigra pars compacta degeneration producing decreased dopamine and increased acetylcholine (ACh)

B. Signs/Symptoms—pill-roll tremor, cogwheel rigidity, bradykinesia, shuffle gait, and mask face

C. Secondary Parkinsonism—olivopontocerebellar degeneration; Shy-Drager syndrome (autonomic dysfunction with orthostatic hypotension); progressive supranuclear palsy (impaired vertical gaze, dysarthria, dysphagia, axial dystonia, emotional lability, survival 6 years); medically induced (Haldol, Compazine, Reglan); lacunes; and trauma.

D. Treatments

1. Dopamine agents—Sinemet with levodopa and carbidopa.

    a. Dopamine does not cross the blood–brain barrier (BBB) but L-dopa does.

    b. Carbidopa (currently the most effective agent) inhibits peripheral decarboxylation of L-dopa and is best for bradykinesia but less effective for tremor.

    c. The major side effect is dyskinesia.

2. Dopamine agonists—bromocriptine (Parlodel).

3. Increase dopamine levels—Eldepryl (MAO-B inhibitor) and amantadine (dopamine agonist; inhibits reuptake)

4. Anticholinesterase—Benadryl (rarely used)

5. Fetal tissue implantation into substantia nigra—questionable benefit

6. Pallidotomy—radiofrequency lesion or stimulator to GPi or subthalamus

    a. Success rates—dyskinesia 90%, bradykinesia 85%, rigidity 75%, tremor 57%

    b. Also improves on/off symptoms.

    c. Complications—visual field cut 3%, hemiparesis, dysarthria 8%, and speech and cognitive decline if bilateral lesions created

7. Thalamotomy—radiofrequency or stimulator to VIM nucleus most effective for tremor.

VI. Acute Disseminated Encephalomyelitis

A. Cause—autoimmune, usually after a viral illness or vaccination

B. Signs/Symptoms—monophasic deterioration with variable deficits that may include altered mentation, weakness, sensory loss, etc.

C. Evaluation—MRI with hyperintense T2 plaque

D. Treatment—steroids

VII. Multiple Sclerosis

A. Cause—demyelination of white matter tracts in the CNS (esp. periventricular)

B. Signs/Symptoms—optic neuritis 50%, internuclear ophthalmoplegia (almost always indicates MS), motor, sensory, and genitourinary

C. Evaluation—two attacks in different places at different times, CSF oligoclonal bands of IgG with normal serum IgG and protein < 100, and MRI plaques (94% specific)

D. Treatment—interferon Beta-1b (Betaseron) injections decrease frequency of attacks by 30%. Steroids of unproven benefit.

VIII. Amyotrophic Lateral Sclerosis

A. Cause—degeneration of alpha motor neurons in the spinal cord and brain stem as well as corticospinal tracts

B. Signs/Symptoms

1. Upper and lower motor neuron dysfunction
2. No cognitive, sensory, or autonomic dysfunction
3. Extraocular muscles and urinary sphincter usually spared
4. Tongue fasciculations common
5. Often lower motor neuron weakness in the legs with a normal MRI

C. Evaluation—clinical and EMG (fibrillations)

D. Survival—4 years

E. Treatment—none

IX. Subacute Combined Systems Disease

A. Cause—vitamin B_{12} deficiency, usually with malnutrition or pernicious anemia

B. Signs/Symptoms—upper and lower motor neuron dysfunction (also may have peripheral neuropathy), impaired bilateral vibratory and touch sensation, and rarely mental or visual deterioration

C. Evaluation

1. CBC to evaluate for macrocytic anemia (MCV > 100) and hypersegmented polymorphonuclear neutrophils (PMNs)
2. MRI may reveal cervical and thoracic posterior and lateral column demyelination.
3. Other tests include B_{12} assay and serum methylmalonic acid and homocysteine.
4. Shilling's test is used to evaluate for pernicious anemia.

D. Treatment—B_{12} injections. Folic acid may correct anemia, but may worsen neurological symptoms.

X. Friedreich's Ataxia

A. Cause—autosomal recessive from chromosome 9

B. Signs/Symptoms

1. Gait ataxia, upper limb motor and sensory loss, and speech disturbances
2. Degeneration of axons and myelin in the posterior columns, corticospinal tracts, and spinocerebellar tracts
3. Degeneration of the cerebellum and brain stem nuclei
4. Motor neurons usually spared
5. Patients tend to have high-arched feet and pes cavus.

C. Evaluation—clinical and MRI with cerebellar and spinal degeneration.

D. Treatment—none. Patients are usually inambulatory 5 years after onset (before 20 years of age) and die by mid-30s.

XI. Acute Transverse Myelitis

A. Cause—cell mediated immunity to CNS by infection, trauma, tumor, or toxin

B. Signs/Symptoms—varied deficits, peaks at 2 days

C. Evaluation—usually hyperintensity on T2 MRI

D. Treatment—steroids (unclear benefit). Fifty percent of patients have a good recovery.

XII. Guillain-Barré Syndrome

A. Cause—possibly an antibody to peripheral myelin causing focal segmental demyelination with acute peripheral neuropathy

B. Signs/Symptoms

1. Usually symmetric weakness, more proximal than distal
2. Little sensory involvement
3. Possible involvement of cranial nerves
4. Possible autonomic dysfunction
5. Onset 3 days to 5 weeks after an upper respiratory infection, surgery, or immunization. Symptoms peak by 4 weeks with recovery over a few weeks after progression stops.

C. Evaluation—CSF with increased protein and normal cells; NCV with prolonged latencies

D. Treatment—plasmapheresis, steroids (not proven helpful), and antibodies (unclear benefit).

E. Differentiate from

1. Acute intermittent porphyria—normal CSF protein, abdominal cramps, urine with δ-aminolevulinic acid
2. Lead poisoning—wristdrop, may be asymmetrical
3. Botulism—descending symmetrical bulbar paresis often with dilated pupils. Normal NCV
   a. Cause—presynaptic impairment of ACh release
   b. Treatment—supportive by managing airway and circulation until toxin leaves system. Antitoxin may be used.

XIII. Myasthenia Gravis

A. Cause—antibodies to nicotinic ACh-receptors on muscles

B. Signs/Symptoms—intermittently weak (at end of day) with diplopia and ptosis in young females and older males

C. Evaluation—CXR (15% have thymoma), collagen panel (other autoimmune diseases common), Tensilon test (endophronium IV or neostigmine improves symptoms), EMG (decreased muscle action potential with repetitive nerve stimulation), and anti-ACh-receptor assay

D. Treatment—anticholinesterase (pyridostigmine, consider decreasing muscarinic side effects with atropine), thymectomy (helps 80% of patients even without thymoma; there is frequent hyperplasia), plasmapheresis, azathioprine (immunosuppressant), and steroids

XIV. Eaton-Lambert (Myasthenic) Syndrome

A. Cause—antibodies to the presynaptic neuromuscular junction preventing ACh release

B. Signs/Symptoms—symmetrical proximal pelvis and shoulder girdle weakness that improves with repetitive activity of the muscles; possible autonomic dysfunction

C. Evaluation—search for primary neoplasm, especially pulmonary oat cell. Only 50% of patients have a known cancer at the time of diagnosis. EMG with incremental response.

D. Treatment—steroids and azathioprine (immunosuppression)

XV. Paraneoplastic Syndrome

A. Cause—unknown, possibly autoimmune (anti-Yo, anti-Hu, etc.).

B. Signs/Symptoms—variable with different parts of CNS and PNS involved; may be acute or subacute and may be purely motor or sensory

C. Evaluation—search for occult malignancy with CXR, etc. CSF to search for cytology and IgG

D. Treatment—steroids

XVI. Meningeal Carcinomatosis

A. Cause—meningeal seeding by tumor cells

B. Signs/Symptoms—headache, multiple cranial neuropathies, CVA, variable symptoms

C. Evaluation—MRI with thickened enhancing leptomeninges; CSF with elevated protein and cells

D. Treatment—steroids, but prognosis dismal

XVII. Polymyositis

A. Cause—autoimmune attack on muscles

B. Signs/Symptoms—proximal symmetrical muscle weakness sparing ocular movements

C. Evaluation—elevated CPK and EMG with fibrillations. Rule out steroid myopathy, myasthenia gravis, hypothyroidism, and hyperparathyroidism.

D. Treatment—steroids

XVIII. Steroid Myopathy—usually symmetrical proximal lower extremity weakness that resoves after steroid discontinued

XIX. Epidural Lipomatosis

A. Cause—accumulation of epidural fat compressing the thoracic spinal cord, usually related to steroids or obesity

B. Signs/Symptoms—back pain, lower extremity weakness, spasticity, sensory loss, and urinary retention or incontinence

C. Evaluation—MRI

D. Treatment—discontinue steroids, weight loss, and rarely thoracic laminectomy with resection of adipose tissue

XX. Neurosarcoid

A. Cause—unknown

B. Signs/Symptoms—cranial neuropathy, hydrocephalus

C. Evaluation—elevated serum angiotensin-converting enzyme (SACE) level 85%, CXR (hilar nodes), and skin biopsy with noncaseating granulomas

D. Treatment—steroids; usually slow recovery

XXI. Fibromuscular Dysplasia

A. Cause—unknown, but possibly a congenital medial defect

B. Signs/Symptoms—headache, vertigo, TIA. Increased incidence of aneurysm (30%), tumor, and dissection

C. Evaluation

1. Angiogram
2. Second-most-common cause of ICA stenosis
3. Eighty percent of cases are bilateral.
4. Most common site is the renal artery, followed by the cervical ICA

D. Treatment—ASA, angioplasty, and resection with reconstruction (difficult)

XXII. Syncope—transient loss of consciousness due to decreased cerebral blood flow

A. Causes

1. Circulatory failure
   a. Impaired vasoconstriction (vasovagal response, postural hypotension, and primary autonomic insufficiency)
   b. Hypovolemia
   c. Decreased venous return (Valsalva's maneuver, coughing, straining)
   d. Decreased cardiac output (dysrhythmia or obstructive)
2. Altered substrate delivery
   a. Hypoxia
   b. Anemia
   c. Hypoglycemia
3. Emotional disturbance

B. Signs/Symptoms

1. Seizures causing sudden loss of consciousness
2. No prodrome, headache, or skin pallor changes
3. Syncopal episodes lack a post-ictal phase.

XXIII. Headaches

A. Differential—hemorrhage, pseudotumor cerebri, meningitis, venous sinus thrombosis, tumor, migraine, sinus disease, ear disease, dental disease, Tolosa-Hunt syndrome

B. Innervation—there is no C1 sensory innervation.

   1. Greater occipital nerve—from C2,3 dorsal rami; provides sensation to the area rostral and medial behind the ear

   2. Lesser occipital nerve—from C2 ventral ramus; provides sensation to the area caudal and lateral behind the ear

   3. Posterior head–neck junction—innervated by the supraclavicular nerve from the C3,4,5 ventral and dorsal rami

C. Migraine

   1. Common—unilateral throbbing headache, nausea, vomiting, photophobia, and no aura of deficit

   2. Classic—includes an aura of focal deficit < 24 h

   3. Complicated—deficit may last up to 30 days

   4. Migraine equivalent—focal deficit without headache

      a. Treatment (acute episode)—Compazine 10 mg IV, Torodol 30 mg IV, sumatriptan SQ, caffeine/ergot 100 mg/1 mg 2 PO. Ergots and triptans are vasoconstrictors.

      b. Prophylaxis—beta-blockers (avoid in asthmatics), calcium-channel blockers, methysergide (seratonin agonist), control of HTN, and avoidance of OCPs.

   5. Other—There is frequently a family history of migraines. Children may present with an acute confusional state.

D. Cluster headaches—unilateral oculofrontal or oculotemporal headaches with ipsilateral conjunctival injection, nasal congestion, rhinorrhea, lacrimation, partial Horner's syndrome, agitation, and flushing (autonomic). Usually in males and last 30 to 90 minutes per day (at similar times) for 4 to 12 weeks with many months of remission

   1. Treatment (acute episode)—100% O_2, ergotamines, sumatriptan, steroids, or radiofrequency sphenopalatine ganglion lesion

   2. Prophylaxis—lithium 300 mg PO t.i.d. and methysergide

E. Pseudotumor cerebri (benign intracranial hypotension)—increased ICP and papilledema without a mass lesion and with a normal CT/MRI. Usually self-limited, though may cause blindness by optic atrophy. Occur most often in overweight females

1. Evaluation—MRI (there may be slit ventricles), LP (ICP $>$ 20 cm water), visual fields (enlarged blind spot and constricted visual fields), CBC, and collagen panel; be sure to rule out venous sinus thrombosis, sarcoid, and lupus erythematosus.

2. Treatment—weight loss, diuretics (acetazolamide or Lasix), steroids, lumboperitoneal shunt (for headaches), or optic nerve sheath fenestration (for visual deterioration).

F. Spontaneous intracranial hypotension—positional headaches exacerbated by standing.

1. Cause—possibly by a tear in a nerve root sleeve.

2. Signs/Symptoms—postural headache exacerbated by standing

3. Evaluation—MRI demonstrates meningeal enhancement. Consider myelography to locate leak.

4. Treatment—bedrest, hydration, Fioricet, NSAIDS, and blood patch; similar to post-LP headaches and should be treated in a similar manner.

XXIV. Temporal Arteritis

A. Cause—autoimmune disease.

B. Signs/Symptoms—headache, eye pain, visual loss (papilledema or optic atrophy, permanent blindness in 7%), jaw claudication

C. Evaluation—elevated erythrocyte sedimentation rate (ESR) and C-reactive protein (CRP) (50% have polymyalgia rheumatica with elevated CPK) and biopsy (granulomatous skip lesions on external carotid artery (ECA) branches and ophthalmic arteries).

D. Treatment—steroids

XXV. Trigeminal Neuralgia

A. Rule out—atypical facial pain, V1 zoster, dental and orbital problems, temporal arteritis, and tumor

B. Etiology—possibly due to ephatic transmission of action potential

C. Signs/Symptoms—lancinating, parazysmal, sharp, electric, facial pain in a trigeminal distribution

D. Evaluation—extra-ocular movements, facial sensation, corneal reflexes, jaw opening (pterygoid) and closing (masseter)

E. Treatment

1. Pharmacological—Tegretol 200 mg t.i.d. [up to 1600 mg/d, may cause confusion and lethargy, low WBC (keep > 3000), SIADH, and elevated liver enzymes], baclofen, Neurontin, and Elavil. Narcotics usually not effective.

2. Surgical

a. Destructive techniques—includes percutaneous balloon gangliolysis; (Fig. 3–1A,B), and glycerol or radiofrequency rhizotomy. The needle for percutaneous techniques is inserted 1 cm from the angle of the mouth, tunneled under the skin inside the cheek, aimed toward the foramen ovale under fluoroscopic guidance along the midpupillary line, and angled toward the zygoma 2 cm from the tragus. The needle should extend to the clivus–petrous ridge on lateral X-ray. Gamma knife radiosurgery is a new option that requires 2 to 6 weeks for improvement in pain. All of the procedures create new numbness as a trade-off for pain relief.

b. Non-destructive technique—microvascular decompression. A vessel (usually by the superior cerebellar artery) compressing the trigeminal nerve is felt to cause emphatic transmission of painful impulses. A small retrosigmoid craniotomy is performed and the vessel is dissected off the nerve which is then insulated with a Teflon pattie. A rare complication is hearing loss; so be sure the patient has contralateral hearing preoperatively. This technique is not usually useful for trigeminal neuralgia related to multiple sclerosis.

XXVI. Glossopharyngeal Neuralgia

A. Signs/Symptoms—lancinating pain into the posterior throat or ear; afferent fibers from the carotid body to the dorsal X brain stem nucleus may cause the heart to stop with the pain.

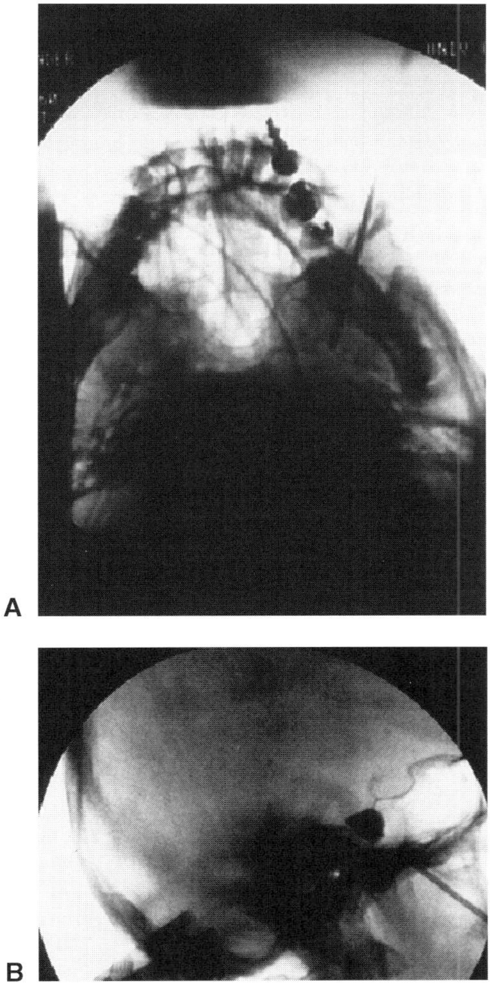

Figure 3–1 (A) Submental skull x-ray with needle in foramen ovale. (B) Lateral skull x-ray with inflated balloon showing characteristic "pear" shape.

B. Treatment

1. Pharmacological—similar to that for trigeminal neuralgia
2. Surgical—consists of craniotomy for microvascular decompression (PICA) or sectioning cranial nerves IX (above the arachnoid fold) and X (only upper two rootlets).

XXVII. Transient Global Amnesia

A. Cause—may be related to migraine or vasospasm

B. Signs/Symptoms—impaired recent and present memory in middle-aged persons; no other symptoms, benign course, seldom recurs

XXVIII. Malignant Neuroleptic Syndrome

A. Causes
   1. Blockage of dopamine receptors in the basal ganglia and hypothalamus after treatment with phenothiazines (Compazine or Thorazine) or Haldol
   2. Possible dysfunction of the muscular sarcoplasmic reticulum
   3. Possible autosomal dominance inheritance
B. Signs/Symptoms—stupor, hyperthermia, hypotension, and rigidity
C. Evaluation—hyperkalemia, myoglobinuria (may cause renal failure), elevated CPK
D. Treatment—bromocriptine (for CNS) and dantrolene (for muscles)

XXIX. Coma

A. Evaluation—electrolytes, CBC, ABG, urine toxicity screen, CT, LP (if CT normal)
   1. Oculovestibular reflex (cold calorics)—do if the tympanic membrane is intact with HOB at 30 degrees. Irrigate 100 mL of ice water in one ear. In an awake patient there should be slow deviation ipsilaterally and the fast nystagmus component contralaterally [cold opposite and warm same (COWS)]. In a comatose patient with a normal brain stem, there should be conjugate ipsilateral deviation but no nystagmus because this requires cortical input.
B. Treatment—consider glucose D50 25 mL, thiamine 100 mg, Narcan, and Romazicon Dilated pupils are usually due to a structural cause, anoxia, or anticholinesterases. Pupils may be dilated with botulism, though the patient is usually awake. Pupils tend to be small with narcotics and pontine lesions.

XXX. Brain Death

A. Signs/Symptoms—pupils fixed and dilated, absent corneal reflexes, oculocephalic reflexes (Doll's eyes), oculovestibular reflexes, gag flexes, and no movement of the body to a painful stimulus (the lower extremities may still have spinal-mediated withdrawal).

B. Evaluation

1. Apnea test

a. Requires $pCO_2 > 60$ mmHg without initiation of a breath.

b. Start with 15 minutes of 100% O_2 and pCO_2 40.

c. Use passive O_2 6 L/min during the test and wait 6 to 12 minutes while maintaining the $pO_2 > 80$.

2. Contributing factors to eliminate

a. T > 32.2°C (90°F)

b. No intoxication

c. Normal O_2

d. SBP > 90

3. Reexamination—usually in 12 hours. For patients 1 year (1 day), 2 months (2 days), neonates (7 days).

4. Confirmation—usually not required. Consider EEG, CBF (radionucleotide angiography), or test with atropine 1 mg (shouldn't affect heart rate because there will be no vagal tone).

XXXI. Weber's Syndrome—cranial nerve III deficit with contralateral hemiplegia

XXXII. Benedikt's Syndrome—Weber's plus red nucleus lesion (ataxia and tremor of UE)

XXXIII. Millard–Gubler Syndrome—cranial nerves VI and VII deficit with contralateral hemiplegia

XXXIV. Parinaud's Syndrome

A. Signs/Symptoms

1. Decreased convergence, accommodation, and upward gaze (setting sun sign, supranuclear dysfunction) with normal vertical Doll's eyes

2. Possible lid retraction, usually caused by a pineal or quadrigeminal plate tumor or elevated ICP with the third ventricle pushing down upon the tectum
3. Differential diagnosis of impaired ocular motility also includes Guillain-Barré syndrome, myasthenia gravis, botulism, Wernicke's encephalopathy, and hypothyroidism.

XXXV. Foster–Kennedy's Syndrome—anosmia, ipsilateral optic atrophy, and contralateral papilledema, usually caused by an olfactory groove meningioma

XXXVI. Dominant Parietal Lobe Lesion—Gerstmann's syndrome with acalculia, agraphia (without alexia), right/left confusion, and finger agnosia

XXXVII. Nondominant Parietal Lobe Lesion—dressing apraxia and neglect (may be from either side)

XXXVIII. Cortical Sensory Syndrome—decreased two-point discrimination, agraphesthesia (draw a number on the palm), and astereognosis (identify a coin in the hand)

XXXIX. Alexia Without Agraphia—usually by a left PCA stroke

XL. Prosoprognosia—due to a lesion in the bilateral or right medial parieto-occipital area

XLI. Superior Vermian Atrophy—trauma, Dilantin, ETOH

XLII. Posterior Column Degeneration—SCSD (B_{12} deficiency), Tabes dorsalis, Freidrich's ataxia.

XLIII. Atonic Bladder—use urecholine to increase ACh. Evaluate with cystometrogram.

XLIV. Spastic Bladder (Hyperreflexic Detrussor)—use ditropan to decrease ACh.

XLV. **Ring-Enhancing Lesion**—vascular, infectious, neoplastic, demyelinating (VIND)

XLVI. **Basal Ganglia Lesions**—infection, astrocytoma, lymphoma, metastatic tumor, demyelination

XLVII. **Suprasellar Mass**—sarcoid, aneurysm/adenoma (pituitary), teratoma, craniopharyngioma, hypothalamic hamartoma/histiocytosis X, meningioma, optic glioma (SATCHMO)

XLVIII. **Sellar Mass**—pituitary adenoma, lymphocytic hypophysitis, sarcoid, TB, pregnancy, and primary hypothyroidism

XLIX. **Transdural Nasal Mass**—juvenile angiofibroma, esthesioneuroblastoma (use chemotherapy before resection and XRT), mucormycosis, meningioma, and metastatic disease

L. **Reversible Posterior Leukoencephalopathy**—demyelination of occipital lobes related to immunosuppression (cyclosporin), hypertension, eclampsia. Usually resolves when the offending agent is withdrawn

LI. **Selective Vulnerability to Hypoxia**—hippocampus (CA1,3), parieto-occipital cortex (layers 3,5), Purkinje cells, outer caudate, and putamen. Likely due to elevated glutamate levels

CHAPTER 4

SEIZURE DISORDERS

I. EVALUATION—electrolytes (hypoglycemia, hyponatremia, hypocalcemia), CBC, CT, LP, toxicology screen, ABG, and EEG.

II. TRAUMATIC

A. Definition—early is < 1 week after injury and late is > 1 week.

B. Treatment—prophylactic anticonvulsants not been proven to decrease late seizure frequency. Use for 3 weeks to 3 months if there is a cortical lesion; then perform EEG before tapering off over 2–4 weeks.

III. STATUS EPILEPTICUS

A. Signs/Symptoms—continuous seizures for > 30 minutes or intermittent without a conscious interval; neurons may be damaged after 20 minutes of firing continuously.

B. Treatment—Ativan 0.1 mg/kg over 2 minutes (or Valium 0.2 mg/kg) and simultaneously load with Dilantin 20 mg/kg IV or phenobarbital 20 mg/kg IV (100 mg/min). If unsuccessful:

1. Consider general anesthesia (always use ABCs); send for electrolytes, glucose, and ABG.
2. Consider giving 50 mL of D50 or thiamine 100 mg IV.

IV. TONIC/CLONIC SEIZURES

A. Treatment—Dilantin, Tegretol, or phenobarbital

V. Absence Seizures

A. Treatment—ethosuximide or valproic acid

VI. Partial Complex Seizures

A. Treatment—Tegretol or Dilantin

VII. Drug Side Effects

A. Dilantin—nystagmus, ataxia, rash, gingival hypertrophy

B. Tegretol—ataxia, SIADH, leukopenia, hepatitis [stop if γ-glutamyltransferase (GGT) 2 × normal].

VIII. Pregnancy

A. Folic acid—use in the first trimester to decrease birth defects

B. Anticonvulsants—increase the risk of congenital malformations; however, persistent seizures carry a higher risk.

IX. Surgery—consider in a patient that has failed 1 year of multidrug therapy

A. Evaluation

1. MRI—look for cortical dysplasia, tumor, or mesial temporal sclerosis
2. Video EEG
3. PET scan—localized hypometabolism ipsilateral to seizure focus in the post-ictal phase
4. Wada's test—assess dominant hemisphere language and memory function with large resection: intracarotid Amytal injection and angiogram to see cross-flow from dominant hemisphere; patient should have a flaccid arm for 5 min.
5. Surgically implanted subdural surface grids—may be used to locate a focus. Avoid intraoperative benzodiazepines and barbiturates; use only narcotics and droperidol. Stimulate the cortex with 60 Hz frequency and 1 volt for 2 msec. Taper the anticonvulsants pre-op and treat

intraoperative seizures with phenobarbital 130 mg IV. After resections, continue anticonvulsants 2 years post-op. Fifty percent of patients become seizure-free, and 80% have decreased frequency after surgery.

B. Resections

1. Anterior temporal lobe—for mesial temporal sclerosis or local lesion

   a. Spare the superior temporal gyrus

   b. Incise the middle temporal gyrus to the temporal horn of the lateral ventricle; dissect over the hippocampus to incisura and choroidal fissure.

   c. Stay subpial to preserve MCA branches.

   d. Resect 5 cm on the dominant side and 7 cm on the nondominant side.

   e. Risks—vessel injury, Meyer's loop injury (contralateral pie-in-sky field cut), and 3rd nerve injury near tentorium

2. Amygdalohippocampectomy

3. Discrete lesionectomy—cortical migration, tumor, or AVM

C. Disconnections—if seizures involve both hemispheres or are from an eloquent location

1. Corpus callosotomy—for drop attacks (atonic seizures)

   a. There is a 70% improvement in seizures.

   b. Cut only the anterior $\frac{2}{3}$ of the corpus callosum to avoid disconnection syndrome (left tactile anomia and dyspraxia, right olfactory anomia and hand spatial problems, decreased spontaneous speech, and incontinence).

   c. Don't cut the anterior commissure.

   d. Consider Wada's test for left-handed patients to avoid language and behavioral problems.

2. Functional hemispherectomy—80% of patients improve.

   a. Leave the basal ganglia intact.

3. Subpial transections—for partial complex seizures in eloquent cortex

   a. Cut every 5 mm to interrupt horizontal spread and leave vertical columns intact.

D. Vagal nerve stimulator—can decrease seizure frequency but does not eliminate seizures. Implant on the left side.

X. EEG Monitoring

A. Helpful in the diagnosis of Creutzfeldt–Jakob disease and subacute sclerosing panencephalitis (SSPE)

B. Can determine burst suppression with barbiturates when used for cerebral ischemia.

C. Intraoperative reversal of SSEP wave helps to localize the motor–sensory strip junction.

   1. An evoked potential decrease in amplitude of 50% or an increase in latency of 10% is considered significant, though there is much debate over how useful this is in surgery with tumor resection.

CHAPTER 5

CEREBROSPINAL FLUID ISSUES

I. RHINORRHEA—CSF may travel from middle ear through eustachian tube to nasopharynx or directly through cribriform plate to nasopharynx

II. OTORRHEA—CSF leak requires perforated tympanic membrane

III. CSF LEAK—increased risk of infection, mainly from streptococcus and staphyloccus, and a mortality $< 10\%$

A. Evaluation

1. CSF fluid glucose—should be > 30 (with tears and mucus it should be < 5)
2. B2-transferrin—found only in CSF
3. Leak site—localize with coronal thin-cut CT of anterior fossa to sella or with CT cisternography with iohexal LP injection followed by Trendelenburg position prone.

B. Treatment

1. Bed rest, stool softeners, acetazolamide (decreases CSF production), and fluid restriction (1500 mL/d)
2. Prophylactic antibiotics—not proven helpful
3. Leak persists > 3 days—place lumbar drain with HOB elevated 10 degrees and drip chamber at shoulder
   a. Avoid tension pneumocephalus—treat by bedrest flat with 100% O_2 and rarely aspiration.

4. Leak persists > 2 weeks or patient develops meningitis—consider surgical intradural repair

IV. Hydrocephalus

A. Evaluation

1. Occipitofrontal circumference
2. CT/MRI
3. Pump shunt
4. Shunt series—skull AP and lateral, chest, and abdominal x-ray
5. Shunt-o-gram
    a. Radionucleotide
    b. 1 mL technetium injection while occluding distal tube
    c. Flush with 3 mL CSF
    d. Immediate abdominal image with gamma camera to rule out distal injection
    e. Image cranium to see proximal patency
    f. Image abdomen in 10 min

B. Treatment

1. Shunts—ventriculoperitoneal, pleural, or atrial
    a. Frontal ventricular access
        i. 1 cm anterior to coronal suture and 3 cm lateral to midline
        ii. Aim catheter toward external acoustic meatus and medial canthus (perpendicular to skull usually works) and insert 5–6 cm
    b. Occipital ventricular access
        i. 7 cm above external occipital protruberance and 3 cm lateral to midline
        ii. Aim catheter toward nasion and insert 10 cm
    c. Ventriculoatrial placement

i. Place occipital burr-hole, sagittal incision over medial sternocleidomastoid

ii. Tunnel between the two incisions, cut down 3 cm proximal to the neck incision

iii. Pass atrial catheter, place ventricular catheter, perform internal jugular stick

iv. Connect tubing after flushing.

2. Third ventriculostomy—to treat aqueductal stenosis
   a. Foramen of Monro—must be 4.5 mm to fit endoscope
   b. Access—same location as for frontal ventricular catheter
   c. Penetrate floor of third ventricle anterior to mamillary bodies and posterior to infundibular and suprachiasmatic recesses
   d. Consider Bugby–Bovie catheter, #3 Fogarty balloon catheter, grasper, and irrigation (Fig. 5–1A–C).
3. Lumboperitoneal shunt—best used for pseudotumor cerebri; shown to increase risk of Chiari malformation in children (70%)
4. Emergent access to ventricles in the office setting—push down optic globe and insert spinal needle through roof of orbit in midpupillary line

C. Complications

1. Malfunction rate—17% in first year; 50% in 5 years, usually by infection or obstruction
2. Craniosynostosis
3. Subdural collections—treat by increasing the valve pressure, adding an antisiphon device, or shunting the subdural space to the peritoneum
4. Visual loss—after shunt placement or with hydrocephalus it may be from PCA occlusion from downward herniation, papilledema, or an enlarged third ventricle compressing the optic chiasm.
5. Slit ventricle syndrome—may be due to overdrainage, intermittent underdrainage, or constant underdrainage
6. Positional headaches relieved by lying down—suggest overdrainage; treat with high valve pressure or antisiphon device
7. Nonpositional headaches—suggest shunt obstruction.

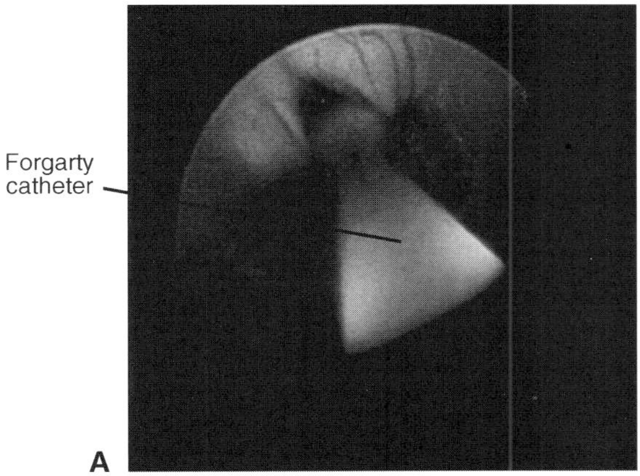

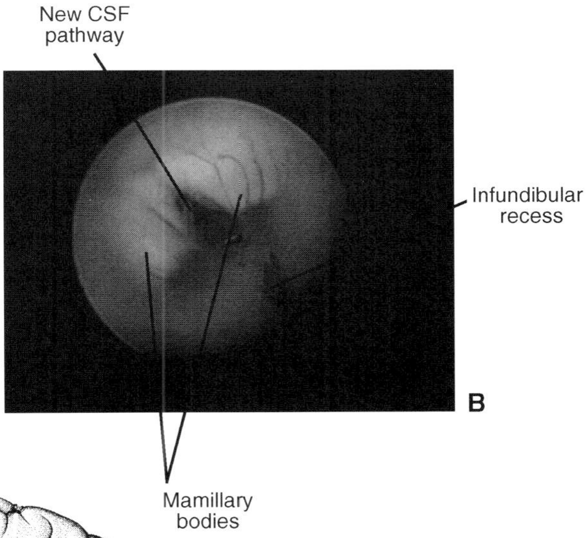

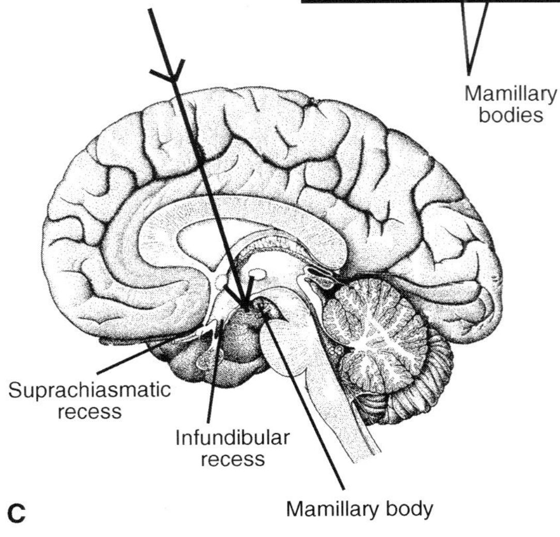

Figure 5–1 (A) Endoscopic view of the floor of the third ventricle with a Fogarty #4 catheter directed into the floor of the ventricle. (B) View after third ventriculocisternostomy. (C) Ventriculostomy anatomy diagram.

8. Ependyma scars and adheres to itself thus allowing increased pressure without a change in ventricular size
9. Shunt unable to be tapped—replace using the same trajectory and consider using an endoscope or image-guided assistance
10. Catheter adheres to choroid or ependyma—remove by inserting a stylet and coagulating with a Bovie

D. Normal-pressure hydrocephalus

1. Signs/Symptoms—apraxic, wide-based gait, urinary incontinence, dementia (impaired memory, usually not severe)
2. Evaluation—CT/MRI and LP (opening pressure > 10 cm water, drain 30 mL to see if patient improves)
3. Treatment—best results for shunting obtained in patients presenting with ataxia
    a. Urinary control improves first.
    b. 35% of patients develop subdural hematoma

CHAPTER 6

INFECTIONS

I. PROPHYLACTIC SURGICAL ANTIBIOTICS

A. Ancef—1 g IV 1 hour before incision and 24 hours postsurgery

B. Vancomycin—if patient allergic to Ancef

C. For nasal or oral surgery—gentamicin 120 mg IV q8h and clindamycin 300 mg IV q8h for 24 hours.

II. MENINGITIS

A. Neonates (< 1 m)—group B strep and *E. coli*

B. Newborns (1–3 m)—strep pneumonia

C. Children (3–7 y)—H. influenza

D. Older children and adults (> 7 y)—N. meningitiditis, *Listeria*

E. Elderly—strep pneumonia

F. Post-op or wound infection—usually staph

G. Chronic meningitis—usually TB, fungus, cysticercosis, tumor, or sarcoid

III. SHUNT INFECTION—50% occur by 2 weeks.

A. Causes—most common organisms are *Staphylococcus epidermidis* and *aureus* and gram-negative rods

B. Signs/Symptoms—fever, leukocytosis, and headache

C. Treatment—externalization of shunt, vancomycin (until cultures back), and shunt replacement after 10 days of antibiotics when CSF is sterile

IV. Laminectomy Infection

A. Cause—usually *S. aureus*. Risk increased in obese, elderly, ill, diabetic, or immunosuppressed.

B. Treatment

1. Culture-guided antibiotics—14 days for superficial infection
2. Surgical debridement
3. Closing over a drain or packing
4. Plastic surgery closure—consider for infection extending down to the bone

V. Skull Osteomyelitis

A. Treatment—3 months of antibiotics; replace bone in 6 months

VI. Brain Abscess

A. Causes—usually strep, fungus (immunocompromised), and gram-negative rods (infants).

B. Evaluation—CBC, ESR, CRP, MRI, Gram stain, culture (also for fungus and AFB).

C. Treatment

1. Antibiotics—6 weeks IV and 6 weeks PO
2. Surgery (to aspirate or excise)—in cases with abscess > 3 cm, unknown organism, location near the ventricle (80% mortality with rupture into ventricle), increased ICP, or failed antibiotic therapy
   a. Use anticonvulsants
   b. Antibiotics may be stopped 1 week after capsule is excised.
   c. Follow-up CTs at 2, 4, and 6 weeks during antibiotic therapy

VII. Subdural Empyema

A. Causes—usually strep and related to recent surgery or adjacent infection

B. Signs/Symptoms—caused by venous thrombosis and infarction

C. Treatment—craniectomy or burr-hole drainage

VIII. Herpes Simplex Virus

A. Signs/Symptoms—hemorrhagic inflammation of medial temporal lobes followed by rapid decline into coma

B. Evaluation

1. MRI—edema
2. LP—increased lymphocytes and protein
3. Biopsy—if unsure of diagnosis; start IV acyclovir before biopsy
4. Polymerase chain reaction—usually returns too late to help

C. Treatment—acyclovir

IX. AIDS—focal lesions are due to Toxoplasma, progressive multifocal leukoencephalopathy (PML), lymphoma, and cryptococcus. There may also be AIDS encephalitis and dementia.

A. Toxoplasmosis

1. Evaluation—detected by a change in baseline titers
2. Treatment—pyrimethamine and sulfadiazine

B. PML

1. Cause—JC virus (JCV)
2. Signs/Symptoms—presents with mental changes
3. Evaluation
   a. MRI with nonenhancing increased T2 signal
   b. Loss of myelin in the white matter
   c. LP may be sent for PCR for JCV.
4. Treatment—none

C. Lymphoma

1. Evaluation—enhances on MRI and is usually near the third ventricle; LP for PCR for EBV.
2. Treatment—radiation and steroids; survival is 3 months.

D. Brain masses

1. Treatment—antitoxoplasma medications for 2 weeks and biopsy if there is no decrease in size

X. Creutzfeldt–Jakob Disease

A. Cause—prion or slow virus

B. Signs/Symptoms—dementia, ataxia, visual loss, and myoclonus

C. Evaluation

1. MRI—hyperintense on T2 in basal ganglia
2. LP—rule out syphilis, may see increased protein
3. EEG—periodic spikes
4. Biopsy—spongiform encephalitis with decreased cells and no inflammation, stain for protease-resistent protein. Sterilize biopsy equipment with steam and sodium hydroxide.

D. Treatment—none; death usually within 1 year

XI. Lyme Disease

A. Cause—*Borrelia burgdorferi*

B. Signs/Symptoms—many symptoms, including bilateral 7th nerve dysfunction. Neurological symptoms are usually preceded by erythema chronicum migrans rash.

C. Evaluation—serum antibody titer

D. Treatment—antibiotics

XII. Cysticercosis

A. Evaluation—serum or CSF ELISA study and CT/MRI

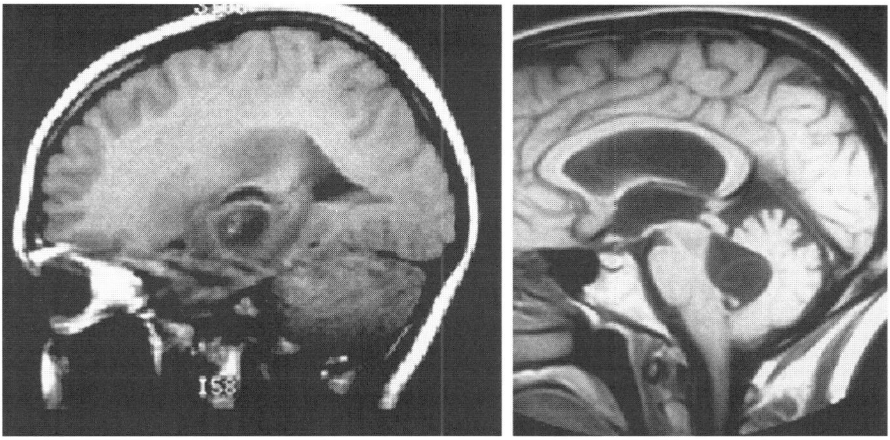

Figure 6–1 Cysticercosis. (A) Noninfused sagittal T1-weighted magnetic resonance images demonstrate cystic lesions with a scolex in the left temporal lobe and (B) in the fourth ventricle. (With permission from Citow JS. Neuropathology and Neuroradiology: A Review. *New York, NY: Thieme Medical Publishers; 2001:30, Fig. 32.)*

B. Treatment

1. Praziquantel or albendazole for 30 days
2. Ocular or spinal cysts—avoid antibiotics
3. Large or intraventricular lesions—consider surgical resection
4. Ventricular shunting—often required (Fig. 6–1A,B)

XIII. Spinal Epidural Abscess

A. Causes—usually due to staph rather than strep. Most often seen in IVDA and diabetics.

B. Signs/Symptoms—pain, tenderness, fever, and focal symptoms related to pressure or thrombophlebitis.

C. Evaluation—MRI, CBC, and ESR.

D. Treatment—antibiotics, immobilization, and decompression.

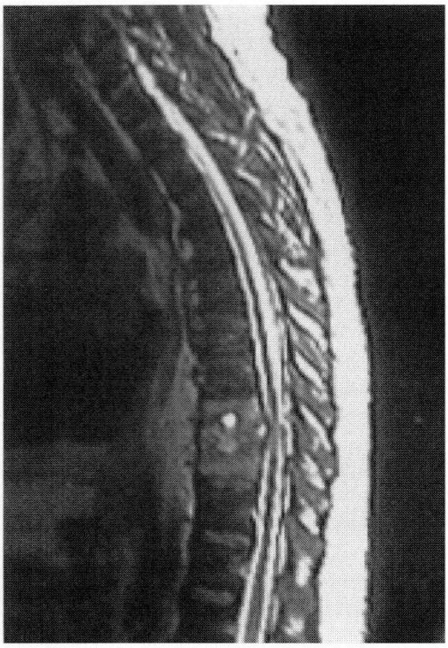

Figure 6–2 T2-weighted magnetic resonance image of the thoracic spine demonstrating Pott's disease with diskitis and osteomyelitis at T7 and 8. (With permission from Citow JS. Neuropathology and Neuroradiology: A Review. *New York, NY: Thieme Medical Publishers; 2001:199, Fig. 272d.)*

XIV. Vertebral Osteomyelitis

A. Causes—usually staph, strep, or TB

B. Treatment—antibiotics and immobilization (Fig. 6–2)

XV. Diskitis

A. Causes—staph and strep

B. Treatment—antibiotics and immobilization

CHAPTER 7

Congenital Lesions

I. Arachnoid Cyst—frequently associated with subdural hematomas

A. Treatment—only if symptomatic

1. Craniotomy and fenestration (consider a shunt if this fails)
2. Consider endoscopic third ventriculostomy and fenestration for a suprasellar cyst.

II. Neurenteric Cyst—lined by gastrointestinal or respiratory endothelium and usually occurs in the cervical or thoracic spine

A. Treatment—resection is required.

III. Encephalocele—most children do not develop normally.

A. Cranial vault (occipital)—most common variety in the Western hemispere

1. Treatment—excision and closing of dura (Fig. 7–1A,B)

B. Sincipital—nasofrontal, nasoethmoidal, and naso-orbital.

C. Basal—transethmoidal, transsphenoidal, sphenoethmoidal, and spheno-orbital. There is no visible mass.

1. Treatment—combination nasal and subfrontal closure

IV. Chiari Malformation

A. Type 1—cerebellar tonsil herniation 5 mm below foramen magnum (varies with age). Presentation is usually around 40 years.

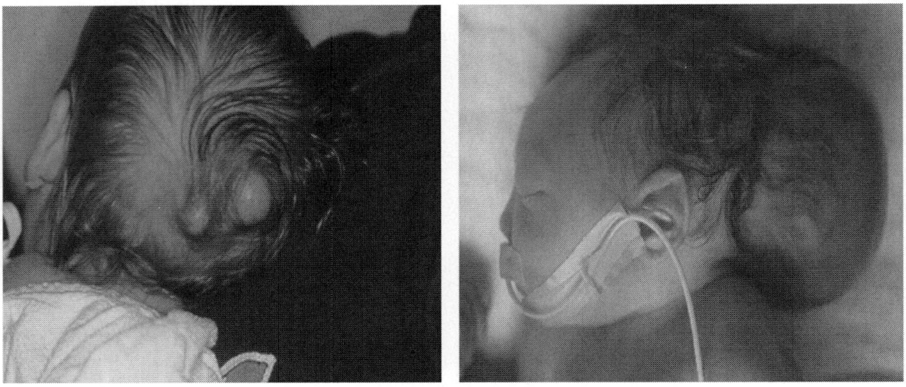

Figure 7–1 Encephaloceles. (A) Two small occipital encephaloceles. (B) Large occipital encephalocele. (With permission from Citow JS. Neuropathology and Neuroradiology: A Review. *New York, NY: Thieme Medical Publishers; 2001:7, Fig. 4.)*

1. Signs/Symptoms—headaches, paresthesias, or syringomyelia
2. Treatment—suboccipital craniectomy and C1 laminectomy with duraplasty (Fig. 7–2)

B. Type 2—always present at birth if the patient has a myelomeningocele (MM).

1. Signs/Symptoms—due to brain stem and cranial nerve dysfunction (dysphagia, stridor, apnea, and nystagmus)
2. Evaluation—MRI shows vermis herniation with tectal beaking, elongated medulla, hydrocephalus, and bony abnormalities
3. Treatment—initially with a ventriculoperitoneal shunt; 20% will eventually require a suboccipital decompression (Fig. 7–3)

V. Dandy–Walker Malformation

A. Cause—atresia of the foramen of Magendie and Luschka with agenesis of the vermis and a posterior fossa cyst communicating with a large fourth ventricle.

B. Signs/Symptoms—associated hydrocephalus (90%) as well as cardiac and multiple other abnormalities. Fifty percent of patients have normal IQs.

C. Treatment—shunting the cyst (Fig. 7–4A–C)

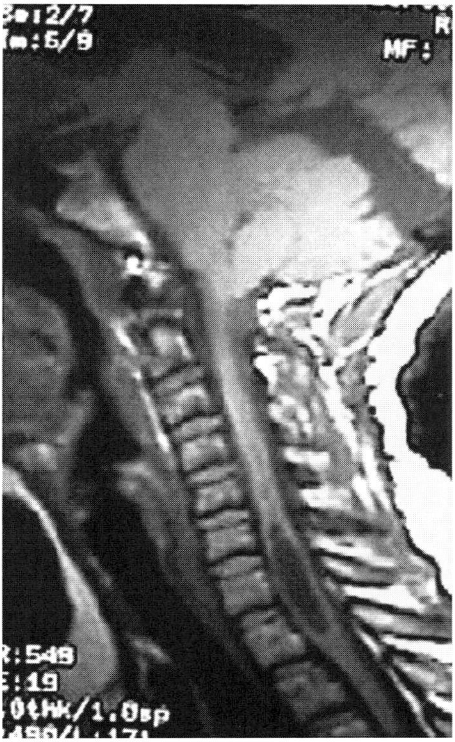

Figure 7–2 Chiari 1 malformation. Sagittal T1-weighted MRI demonstrates peglike tonsils extending below foramen magnum with an associated syrinx. (With permission from Citow JS. Neuropathology and Neuroradiology: A Review. *New York, NY: Thieme Medical Publishers; 2001:13, Fig. 11.)*

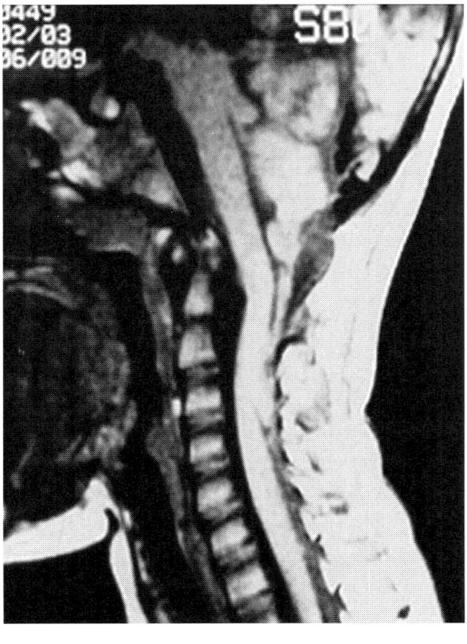

Figure 7–3 Chiari 2 (Arnold-Chiari) malformation. Sagittal T1-weighted MRI with tectal beaking, low-lying torcula, and vermian descent. (With permission from Citow JS. Neuropathology and Neuroradiology: A Review. *New York, NY: Thieme Medical Publishers; 2001:13, Fig. 12.)*

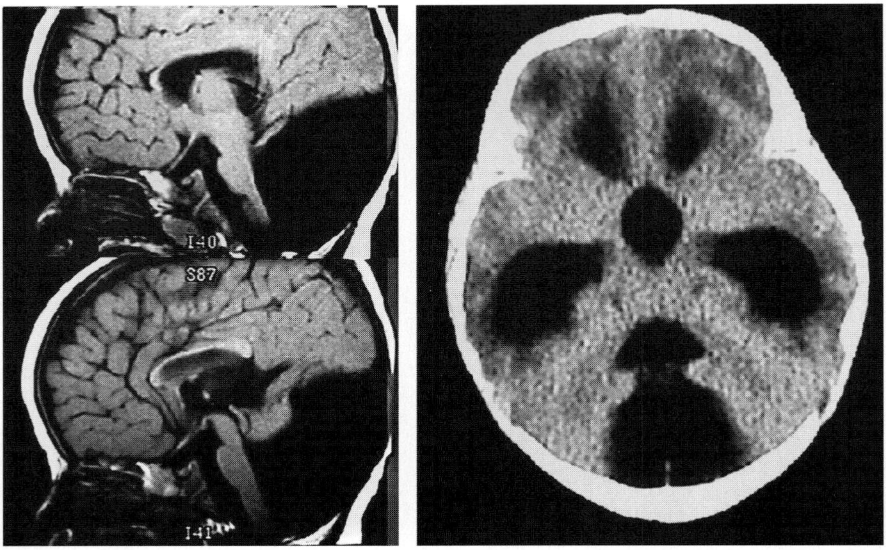

Figure 7–4 Dandy–Walker malformation. (A,B) Sagittal T1-weighted MRIs and (C) axial CT demonstrate vermian agenesis and connection of fourth ventricle to posterior fossa cyst. (With permission from Citow JS. Neuropathology and Neuroradiology: A Review. *New York, NY: Thieme Medical Publishers; 2001:15, Fig. 15.)*

VI. Aqueductal Stenosis

A. Treatment—VP shunt or third ventriculostomy

VII. Myelomeningocele (Fig. 7–5A,B)

A. Facts—Eighty percent have hydrocephalus, most have Chiari 2 malformation, 80% have normal IQ, and 10% have normal urinary continency.

B. Prevention

1. Folic acid supplements during the first trimester
2. Avoid valproic acid, saunas, and hot tubs in the first trimester.

C. Evaluation

1. 3% risk after a prior abnormal birth
2. Maternal serum alpha fetal protein (AFP), ultrasound, and amniocentesis for AFP

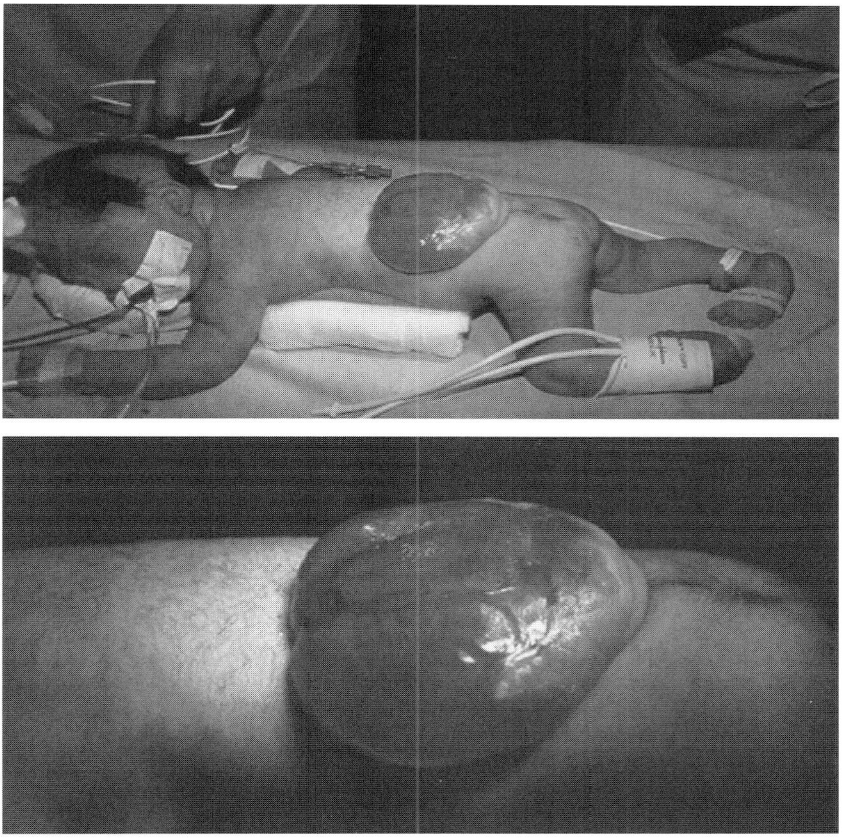

Figure 7–5 Myelomeningocele. (A) Neural placode noted on center of dorsal aspect. (B) Close-up image. (With permission from Citow JS. Neuropathology and Neuroradiology: A Review. *New York, NY: Thieme Medical Publishers; 2001:7, Fig. 3.)*

3. Evaluate the child for spontaneous leg movement, scoliosis, hip and knee abnormalities (x-rays).
4. GU evaluation—15% have abnormalities such as one kidney or a horseshoe kidney; perform a straight catheterization.
5. Cardiac echo—15% have abnormalities such as atrial or ventricular septal defects.
6. Head ultrasound—most have hydrocephalus.

D. Treatment—85% survival

1. Cover the lesion with Telfa and sponges soaked with normal saline (consider connecting IV tubing running at 5 mL/h to the gauze)
2. Maintain prone Trendelenburg position.
3. If ruptured, use nafcillin and gentamicin until 6 h after closure.
4. If unruptured don't use antibiotics.
5. Closure within 24 hours.
6. If no hydrocephalus by ultrasound and occipital-frontal circumference (OFC) measurements, repair the MM and shunt in 3 days if needed.
7. If there is hydrocephalus, operate in the prone position with the head turned.
   a. Shunt the ventricles to the peritoneum via the flank
   b. Begin MM repair by isolating the placode and removing the tissue between the placode and skin.
   c. Suture the cord into a cylinder.
   d. Close the dura, fascia, and skin.
   e. Complications include shunt malfunction, syrinx, and tethered cord.
   f. There is no proof that birth by C-section alters outcome.

VIII. Lipomyelomeningocele—skin-covered lesion

A. Signs/Symptoms—most have cutaneous stigmata of spina bifida such as a hair patch, dimple, or red mark.

B. Evaluation—MRI

C. Treatment

1. Untether the cord and debulk the fat
2. Use intraoperative SSEP and nerve root stimulation.
3. Surgical outcome—unchanged (75%), improved (20%), worse (5%)

IX. Dermal Sinus Tract

A. Signs/Symptoms

1. Cutaneous indication is a dimple with hair
2. Often meningitis

B. Evaluation—MRI and x-ray (to find spina bifida)

C. Treatment—repair with resection of tract and dural closure.

X. Tethered Cord—low-lying conus below L2 with thickened filum or mass; frequently associated with MM; cutaneous manifestations in 50%

A. Signs/Symptoms—gait dysfunction (90%), sensory loss (70%), bladder dysfunction (40%), scoliosis, pain

B. Evaluation—cystometrogram, x-ray (spina bifida is seen in 98%), MRI

C. Treatment—stimulate the filum before sectioning.

1. Filum terminale is whiter than the nerve roots and has ligamentous fibers with a squiggly vessel on the surface.
2. Intraoperative anal sphincter EMG

XI. Diastematomyelia—spinal cord split into two longitudinal sections

A. Treatment—remove the bony interspinal bar and untether the filum.

XII. Klippel-Feil Syndrome—congenital fusion of at least two cervical vertebrae; associated with multiple systemic anomalies (one kidney, cardiac irregularities, etc.).

A. Evaluation—EKG, CXR, and renal ultrasound.

B. Treatment

1. Fuse from an anterior and posterior approach if unstable after trauma

XIII. Craniosynostosis

A. Fontanelles—anterior closes at 18 months; posterior closes at 3 months.

B. Skull diploë—forms at 4 years in unilaminar bone

C. Evaluation

1. Palpate the prominent suture.
2. X-ray may fail to demonstrate a normal lucent suture.
3. 3-D CT reconstruction demonstrates the abnormal shape.

D. Sagittal synostosis—most common variety; more often seen in males

1. Signs/Symptoms—dolichocephalic or scaphocephalic shape with decreased biparietal distance.
2. Treatment
    a. Prone position with a strip craniectomy from coronal suture to lambdoid suture 3 cm wide at 3 to 6 months.
    b. Skull remodeling—required after 1 year to make the skull shorter and wider
    c. Be careful about blood loss and hypothermia.

E. Coronal synostosis—more common in females

1. Unilateral—plagiocephaly
    a. Normal side bulges; abnormal side has a harlequin eye due to elevated supraorbital margin (Fig. 7–6)
2. Bilateral—brachycephaly with proptosis and maxillary hypoplasia

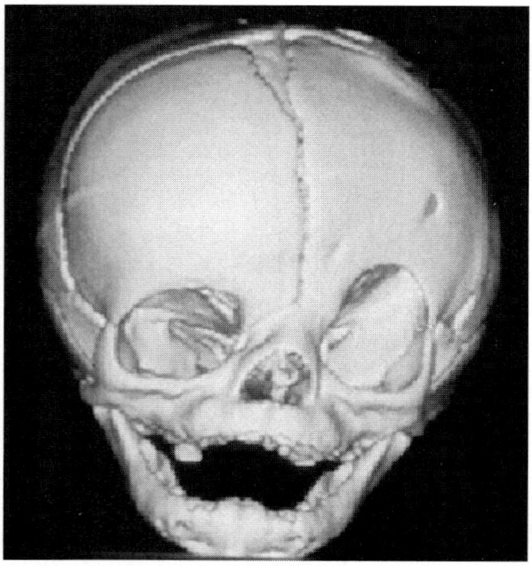

Figure 7–6 Unilateral coronal synostosis (plagiocephaly). CT reconstruction with harlequin eye on the left. (With permission from Citow JS. Neuropathology and Neuroradiology: A Review. *New York, NY: Thieme Medical Publishers; 2001:17, Fig. 17.)*

3. Crouzon's syndrome—bilateral synostosis with midface hypoplasia of sphenoid, orbital, and facial bones
4. Apert's disease—as with Crouzon's syndrome syndactyly, hydrocephalus, low IQ
5. Treatment—strip craniectomy or frontal craniotomy with lateral canthal advancement at 3 to 6 months with absorbable plates

F. Metopic synostosis—trigonocephaly

G. Lambdoid synostosis—more common in males and on the right side

1. Evaluation—rule out positional plagiocephaly due to the child lying on one side too much.
2. Treatment—molding helmet (if positional) or strip craniectomy at 6 to 18 months

CHAPTER 8

Functional Neurosurgery

I. Parkinsonism

A. Treatment

1. Thalamotomy—VIM nucleus to treat tremor
2. Pallidotomy—GPi lesion to treat rigidity or bradykinesia. Also useful for levodopa-induced dyskinesias and on–off problems
3. Stimulation—of thalamus, globus pallidus, or subthalamic nucleus
4. Surgery—avoid if the patient has dementia, a coagulation disorder, contralateral hemianopsia, or secondary parkinsonism
5. Remember to create a lesion contralateral to the symptomatic side.
    a. 80% of patients are improved.
    b. Microelectrode recording helps determine the location of the radiofrequency lesion.
6. Complications—visual field cut, hemiparesis, blood clot, and dysarthria (especially if bilateral)

II. Spasticity

A. Treatment

1. Medical
    a. Prolonged stretching to decrease contractures
    b. Valium

c. Baclofen

d. Dantrolene

2. Surgical

a. Intrathecal baclofen

b. Neurectomy or blocks

c. Radiofrequency rhizotomy or open selective dorsal rhizotomies—EMG intra-op

d. Midline thoracic myelotomy with T11–L1 laminectomy—cut the T12–S1 cord to spare the S2–4 bladder reflex 4 mm deep.

III. Torticollis

A. Cause—dystonia by spasm of the sternocleidomastoid muscle

B. Evaluation—rule out C1–2 rotatory subluxation, 11th nerve compression, infection, or tumor.

C. Treatment—physical therapy, TENS unit, spinal cord stimulator, BoTox injection, section spinal accessory nerve (XI), or microvascular decompression of XI from the vertebral artery.

IV. Hemifacial Spasm

A. Cause—compression of VII by the anterior inferior cerebellar artery (AICA) at the root entry zone (REZ)

1. Compression of VIII causes tinnitus.

2. Brain stem glioma or multiple sclerosis can cause facial myokymia (continuous facial spasm).

3. Blepharospasm is bilateral eyelid spasms.

B. Treatment—BoTox injections or a microvascular decompression

V. Hyperhidrosis—increased sweating (esp. in the palms)

A. Evaluation—rule out hyperthyroidism, diabetes, pheochromocytoma, Parkinson's disease, and menopause.

B. Treatment—antiperspirants, anticholinesterases, or sympathectomy

VI. Sympathectomy—used to treat hyperhidrosis, Raynaud's syndrome, angina, or reflex sympathetic dystrophy (RSD).

1. For upper extremity symptoms—remove the sympathetic ganglia at T2 (to avoid Horner's syndrome) via an open midline T3 costotransversectomy or thoracoscopic approach.

VII. Chronic Pain

A. Conservative management options—physical therapy, oral medications (NSAIDs, steroids, Elavil, Neurontin, narcotics), and epidural steroid injections

B. Deep brain stimulation—placed in the periaqueductal or periventricular gray

C. Spinal cord stimulator—for RSD, failed back syndrome, arachnoiditis, and refractory angina.

   1. Place the electrodes percutaneously (Pieces) or open (Resume) and connect to an internal pulse generator.

D. Intrathecal pumps

   1. May use SQ reservoir or pump (if $>$ 3-month survival)
   2. Test with 2 mg CSF injection
      a. Watch for decreased breathing $<$ 10/min and have Narcan 0.4 mg ready (1 amp)
         i. Intrathecal dose—$\frac{1}{10}$ the epidural dose, $\frac{1}{100}$ the IV dose, and $\frac{1}{300}$ the oral dose.
         ii. Bolus 0.4 mg post-op
   3. 90% have significantly improved pain control.

E. Cordotomy—useful for cancer pain involving one limb or one side of the body.

   1. Performed on the side contralateral to the pain because the crossed lateral spinothalamic tract is severed.
   2. C1–2 percutaneous method usually used with fluoroscopic guidance.

3. Needle should be anterior to the dentate ligament.
4. Open procedure may be done in the thoracic spine.
5. Complications—ipsilateral weakness, urinary incontinence, and Ondine's curse (failure of involuntary respiration with bilateral cervical procedures)

F. Midline myelotomy—for bilateral pain below the thoracic region
1. After laminectomy, the midline sulcus is penetrated with a Penfield #4 down to the central canal extending from T10 to two levels above the conus (to avoid bladder dysfunction).

G. Hypophysectomy—for severe bone pain related to breast or prostate cancer
1. May be performed with radiosurgery, open resection, or insertion of alcohol

H. Cingulotomy—for diffuse pain; a last resort

I. Dorsal root entry zone (DREZ) lesion—for deafferentation pain due to nerve root avulsion.

VIII. Reflex Sympathetic Dystrophy (Complex Regional Pain Syndrome, Causalgia)

A. Cause—unknown

B. Signs/Symptoms
1. Burning pain—usually in the median, ulnar, and sciatic nerves
2. Vasomotor changes—pink or cold and with increased or decreased sweating
3. Trophic changes—dry and thin skin, stiff joints, possibly due to immobility

C. Evaluation—clinical and with sympathetic blocks; NCV may be useful to rule out nerve compression

D. Treatment
1. Physical therapy—most useful option, with muscle stretching
2. Elavil, Neurontin, phentolamine IV

3. Stellate ganglion block—better at T2 to avoid Horner's syndrome
4. Lumbar sympathetic blocks
5. Surgical sympathectomy
6. Spinal cord stimulator

CHAPTER 9

TUMORS

I. RADIATION—avoid in children < 5 years old; consider chemotherapy until CNS becomes more developed

II. LOW-GRADE ASTROCYTOMA

A. Treatment

1. Usually with surgery alone (esp. with juvenile pilocytic astrocytoma)
2. Radiation dose, if used—45 Gy to the tumor with a 2 cm margin
3. Chemotherapy—procarbazine, CCNU, and vincristine (PCV).

III. HIGH-GRADE ASTROCYTOMA

A. Prognosis—depends on age (younger is better), Karnofsky score, and histology.

B. Treatment

1. Cytoreductive surgery—image-guided surgery suggested
2. External beam radiation—40 Gy to the whole brain and 20 Gy to the tumor bed
3. PCV chemotherapy
4. Gliadel (BCNU) wafers—increase survival by 8 weeks (Lancet 1995).
5. Temodar—an oral alkylating agent that may help a little.
6. Surgery—avoid if tumor is in dominant hemisphere or is bilateral, or in patients with low Karnofsky score

C. Survival

1. Per grade—1 (10 y), 2 (8 y), 3 (2 y), and 4 (< 1 y)
2. Average—17 weeks with biopsy, 30 weeks with surgery

IV. Oligodendroglioma

A. Treatment—surgery, chemotherapy (PCV helps significantly), XRT (for the anaplastic variety).

B. Survival—30% at 10 years

V. Ependymoma

A. Evaluation—evaluate for drop mets with LP and spinal MRI.

B. Treatment

1. Surgery
2. XRT—50 Gy to the tumor bed, and spinal XRT if drop mets are seen or cells detected in the CSF

C. Survival—tumor is usually very radiosensitive; survival is 40% at 5 years in children, 80% at 5 years in adults

VI. Choroid Plexus Tumors

A. Treatment—surgery only; consider preoperative embolization

VII. Primitive Neuroectodermal Tumor (PNET)

A. Evaluation—evaluate for drop mets with spinal MRI and LP.

B. Treatment

1. Surgery
2. XRT—radiate craniospinal axis after resection, after 3 years in children
3. Modest surgical resection for medulloblastoma

a. Craniospinal XRT—40 Gy with 15 Gy to the tumor bed and drop mets over 6 weeks

b. Chemotherapy—CCNU and vincristine

4. Shunt—required in 30% of cases

C. Survival—tumor is usually very radiosensitive; survival is 43% in 10 years.

VIII. Ganglioglioma

A. Treatment—surgery alone

IX. Pineal Tumors—pineal region borders are the tectum, vermis, splenuim of the corpus callosum (posteriorly), third ventricle (superiorly), and thalami (laterally).

A. Evaluation

1. Evaluate for drop mets with all varieties.

2. Tumor varieties

a. Germ cell—most common; most often germinoma

b. Pineocytoma/pineoblastoma, astrocytoma, embryonal carcinoma, choriocarcinoma, and teratoma

3. CSF for AFP—in embryonal carcinoma, endodermal sinus tumor, and teratoma

4. BHCG—choriocarcinoma and germinoma

B. Treatment

1. If tumor resection does not relieve hydrocephalus—place VP shunt or perform third ventriculostomy (penetrate floor of third ventricle anterior to mamillary bodies).

2. Avoid performing a stereotactic biopsy due to the hazard of adjacent vessels.

3. Germinoma may be treated with biopsy followed by radiation and chemotherapy.

4. Resection carries a 10% mortality.

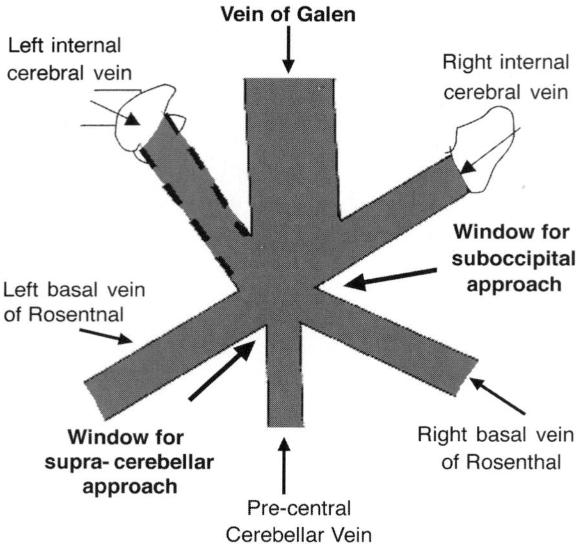

Figure 9–1 Surgical windows around the deep venous anatomy for pineal region lesions.

C. Operative approaches

1. Infratentorial/supracerebellar
    a. Not as easy with a steep tentorium
    b. Usually safe to divide the precentral cerebellar vein
    c. Operative window—between the two basal veins of Rosenthal (Fig. 9–1)
2. Suboccipital/transtentorial
    a. Risks visual loss
    b. Best for tumors above the tentorial edge and vein of Galen (Fig. 9–2A,B)
    c. Incise the tentorium 1 cm lateral to the straight sinus.
    d. Operative window—between internal cerebral vein and basal vein of Rosenthal
3. Transcallosal
4. Transventricular—through the superior temporal gyrus

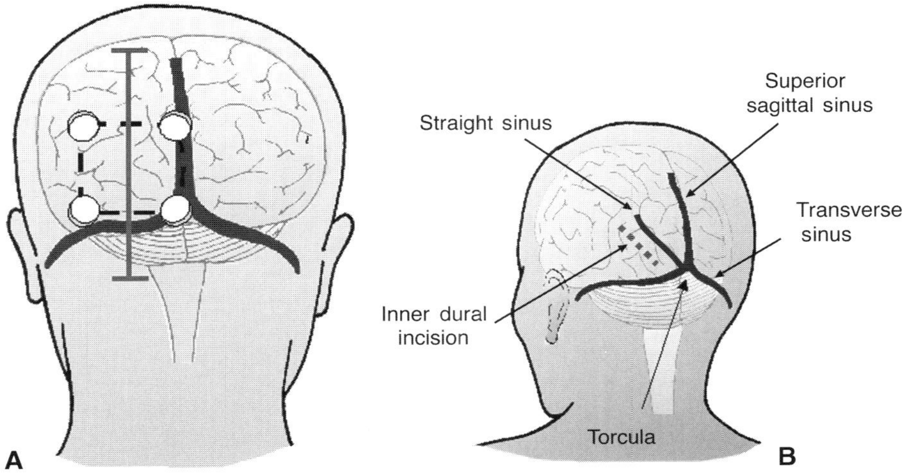

Figure 9–2 (A) Suboccipital and (B) transtentorial incision.

X. Pituitary Adenoma

A. Apoplexy

1. Signs/Symptoms—typically presents with headache and ophthalmoplegia
2. One third of prolactin-secreting adenomas will hemorrhage
3. Not an emergency if asymptomatic
4. Treatment in cases with mass effect—steroids and surgical decompression

B. Signs/Symptoms

1. Bitemporal hemianopsia
2. Cavernous sinus invasion—impaired cranial nerves III–VI, chemosis, proptosis, and rarely CVA
3. Hypo- or hyperpituitarism
   a. Increased prolactin
      i. Amenorrhea, galactorrhea, and impotence
      ii. May also be seen with hepatic or renal disease, phenothiazines, verapamil, cimetidine, and pregnancy

b. Increased adrenocorticotropic hormone (ACTH)—increased serum and urine cortisol, hyperpigmentation (Nelson's syndrome), hypertension, hyperglycemia, abdominal stria, moon face, truncal obesity, extremity wasting, bruising, osteoporosis, amenorrhea, peripheral neuropathy, and depression

c. Decreased ACTH—orthostatic hypotension and fatigue

d. Increased growth hormone (GH)

   i. Increased somatomedin C—synthesized in the liver and produces IGF-1

   ii. Acromegaly—coarse facial features, enlarging hat size, and enlarging hands and feet

   iii. Peripheral neuropathy, cardiomyopathy, hypertension, glucose intolerance (diabetes), upper airway obstruction, perspiration, colon cancer, and giantism (if occurs before growth plate closes)

   iv. Somatostatin decreases GH release.

e. Decreased GH—dwarfism

f. Decreased thyroid stimulating hormone (TSH)—cold intolerance, fatigue, coarse hair, peripheral neuropathy, and myxedema coma

g. Decreased FSH/LH—amenorrhea, decreased libido, and infertility (hypogonadism)

h. Decreased anti-diuretic hormone (ADH)—diabetes insipidus (very rare with a sellar mass)

C. Evaluation

1. Endocrine history (as above), visual fields, extraocular movements

2. Prolactin—mild elevation to 25–150 is usually by stalk effect from decreased dopamine that normally inhibits prolactin

3. Morning cortisol, 24-hour urine cortisol

4. ACTH—decreased with adrenal tumor, increased with pituitary adenoma or ectopic lung mass

5. Dexamethasone suppression test

   a. Low dose of 1 mg—normally decreases ACTH

   b. High dose of 8 mg—decreases ACTH with Cushing's disease (pituitary adenoma)

   c. There is no suppression with an ectopic tumor

6. TSH, T4, GH, somatomedin C, FSH/LH, estrogen, testosterone
7. MRI
   a. May be normal in 50% of cases
   b. Enlarged pituitary gland on MRI
      i. May be caused by pregnancy (also with amenorrhea and increased prolactin)
      ii. May be caused by primary hypothyroidism (elevated TSH, treat with synthroid)
8. Petrosal sinus sampling—has been used to evaluate the location of an ACTH-secreting tumor; however, normal people have different amounts of ACTH on each side.
9. Rapid-sequence infused MRI—may demonstrate location of a small adenoma.

D. Treatment

1. Prolactinoma
   a. Bromocriptine (Parlodel)—dopamine agonist that decreases tumor size 75% by 8 weeks
   b. Lifelong therapy needed to control tumor growth
   c. Starting dose—2.5 mg PO t.i.d.
   d. Initial bothersome side effects—emesis and postural hypotension; normally resolve over several weeks
   e. Watch for low estrogen—may cause osteoporosis
   f. Safe to take oral contraceptives (OCP) with bromocriptine and safe to take bromocriptine while pregnant
   g. If tumor enlarges during pregnancy, surgically resect it or increase the bromocriptine.
   h. Follow patient with visual field examinations
   i. Dostinex is another medical option.
   j. Consider transsphenoidal or subfrontal resection if medical therapy fails.

2. Acromegaly
   a. Surgical resection—best option, followed by therapy with bromocriptine or octreotide, and finally XRT.
   b. Post-op steroid withdrawal is a good sign.
   c. IGF-1 levels usually drop 4 weeks after surgery.
   d. Tumors with growth hormone levels > 40 are difficult to cure.
3. Cushing's disease
   a. Surgical resection—best option
   b. Ketoconazole may be used to temporarily lower cortisol levels.
   c. Bilateral adrenalectomy—last resort (patient may develop Nelson's syndrome)
4. Hyperthyroidism—surgical resection favored over octreotide
5. Radiation
   a. 50 Gy over 6 weeks
   b. 50% decrease in ACTH, FSH/LH, and TSH in 10 years
   c. Visual loss may occur.
   d. Consider only if unable to reoperate
6. Surgery—subfrontal or transsphenoidal
   a. Transnasal transsphenoidal—most common approach
      i. Insert a throat pack, prep the thigh for a fat graft, inject the nasal mucosa with epinephrine, enter the right nostril
      ii. In a submucosal plane dissect the left side of the nasal cartilage and bilateral nasal bone to the sphenoid bone (find the sphenoid osteum at the top of the exposure)
      iii. Insert the Cushing speculum and finally the Hardy speculum, assess the midline (sphenoid ridge may be off-center), chisel off the floor of the sphenoid sinus, remove the mucosa
      iv. Chisel off the floor of the sella, incise the dura, and curette out the soft tumor.
      v. A newer approach is to insert the speculum directly to the floor of the sphenoid sinus, open the speculum to displace the nasal

bone, and open the mucosa over the sinus wall and proceed from there.

vi. Lumbar drain may be inserted and air injected to help push the tumor down during resection.

vii. Post-op MRI should be done at 3 months.

E. Complications

1. Diabetes insipidus (DI), injuries to cranial nerves II–VI, carotid artery injury, hypopituitarism, and CSF leak.
2. Antibiotics—use until the packs are removed at 3 days (chloramphenicol and ampicillin) as well as a hydrocortisone stress dose followed by a replacement dose (100 mg IV q8h × 3 then 20 mg PO qAM and 10 mg qHs).
3. Hydrocortisone—stop 2 days after surgery and send a urine cortisol (< 9 needs steroid replacement).
4. Diabetes insipidus—diagnosed as a urine output (UOP) > 250 mL/h × 3 hours with specific gravity (SG) < 1.005.
5. Lost fluid—replace with $\frac{1}{2}$ NS and use 0.1 μg DDAVP IV q6h or intranasal 10–40 μg b.i.d. for long-term maintenance.
6. CSF leak—treat initially with a lumbar drain and if this is unsuccessful, consider exploration and packing.
7. Carotid injury with pulsatile bleeding—should be treated with packing followed by an angiogram to determine if bypass or endovascular treatment (occlusion, stenting, etc.) is needed.

XI. Craniopharyngioma

A. Treatment

1. Perform pre-op and post-op endocrine evaluation.
2. Steroids—use as in Section X. E. 3 after surgery.
3. Subtotal resection—appears to be the best treatment (unless complete removal can be safely achieved), followed by XRT
4. Surgical approach—usually subfrontal
5. Surgical mortality—10%; morbidity includes hyperthermia, lethargy, impaired thirst mechanism, and endocrine deficiencies.

B. Survival—5-year is 75%.

XII. Colloid Cyst

A. Treatment

1. If < 7 mm and without hydrocephalus, consider conservative management with follow-up MRI at 6 months.
2. Surgical management—stereotactic aspiration or open transcallosal resection (remember to fenestrate the septum pellucidum)
3. Surgical pitfalls—damage to the internal cerebral veins and fornix

XIII. Meningioma

A. Treatment

1. Surgical resection—consider if symptomatic
   a. Pre-op—remember to consider dural patch material (autograft or synthetic), dural sinus patency, and possibility of embolization (may however cause distant strokes).
   b. Recurrence with partial resection—60% at 10 years without XRT; 30% with XRT.

B. Survival—91% at 5 years

XIV. Vestibular Schwannoma

A. Evaluation—should include pure tone audiogram and speech discrimination test (50/50 is considered serviceable hearing with 50 Db pure tone hearing and 50% speech discrimination).

B. Treatment—if asymptomatic, consider following with MRI evaluation every 6 months (Fig. 9–3A,B).

1. Suboccipital retrosigmoid resection
2. Middle fossa approach—for small intracanalicular tumors distal in the canal
3. Translabyrinthine approach—sacrifices hearing

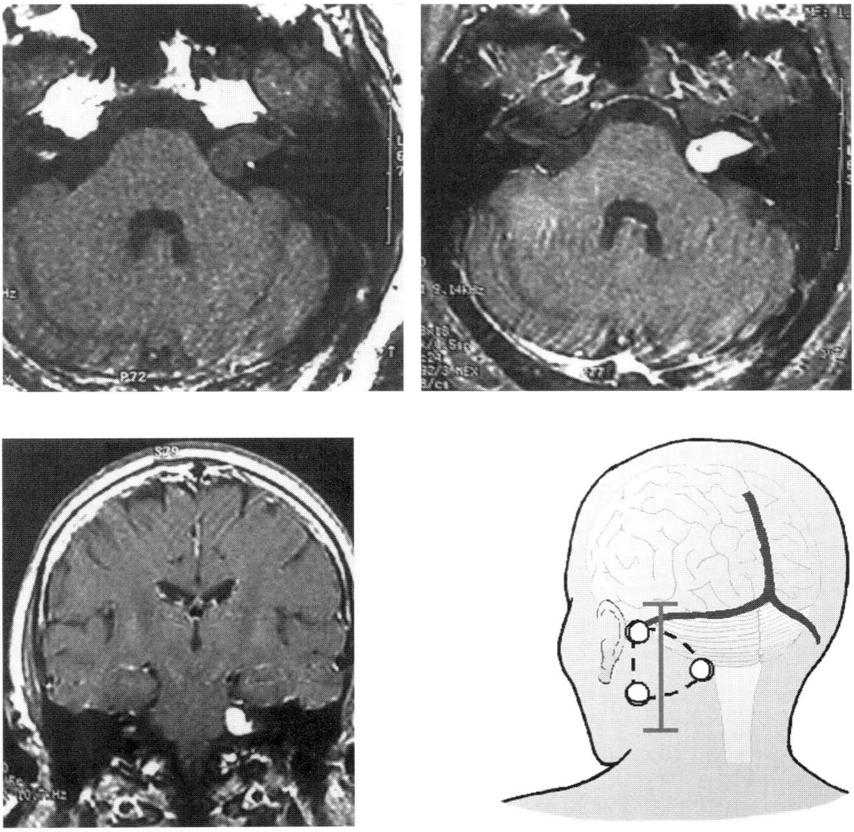

Figure 9–3 (A) Vestibular schwannoma, noninfused, (B) infused, and (C) axial and infused coronal T1-weighted magnetic resonance images demonstrating an enhancing mass emanating from the left internal acoustic meatus. (With permission from Citow JS. Neuropathology and Neuroradiology: A Review. *New York, NY: Thieme Medical Publishers; 2001:105, Fig. 147.) (D) Vestibular schwannoma exposure via suboccipital–retrosigmoid craniotomy.*

4. XRT/stereotactic radiosurgery—14 Gy dose, undetermined indication with primary or recurrent tumors, and associated with lower hearing preservation and increased risk of facial palsy
5. Use intra-op 8th (BAER), 7th, and 5th nerve monitoring.
6. Suboccipital retrosigmoid craniotomy
    a. Place the patient semi-prone (45 degrees) or lateral with the falx parallel to the floor.

b. Incision is the length of the pinna and located 2 cm posterior to the mastoid notch.

c. A burr hole is made at the asterion and a small craniotomy fashioned.

d. Dura is opened with triangular flaps based on the transverse and sigmoid sinuses.

e. Cerebellum is gently and slowly retracted medially to expose the cranial nerves.

f. Water-tight dural closure is essential.

g. Complications

i. Facial palsy—if unable to close eyes, use natural tears q2h, Lacrilube, and tape eye shut qHs

ii. Tarsorrhaphy—if after 1 year the weakness hasn't improved, perform a XII–VII anastomosis (or even after only 2 months if the nerves were directly cut)

iii. CSF leak—treat with a lumbar drain, shunt, or ENT packing

iv. Vertigo—resolves with rehab

C. Preservation of function

1. Seventh nerve—95% (< 1 cm), 80% (1–2 cm), 50% (> 2 cm)

2. Eighth nerve—57% (< 1 cm), 33% (1–2 cm), 6% (> 2 cm)

XV. Trigeminal Schwannoma—much less common than vestibular schwannoma.

A. Tumor limited to Meckel's cave in the middle fossa—pterional craniotomy should provide sufficient exposure.

B. Dumbbell-shaped tumor with extension into the posterior fossa—more aggressive approach such as the transpetrosal

C. Dissection may be epidural (find V2 and V3 and trace to the tumor) or intradural (Fig. 9–4).

XVI. Hemangioblastoma—usually located in the posterior fossa near the sigmoid–transverse junction.

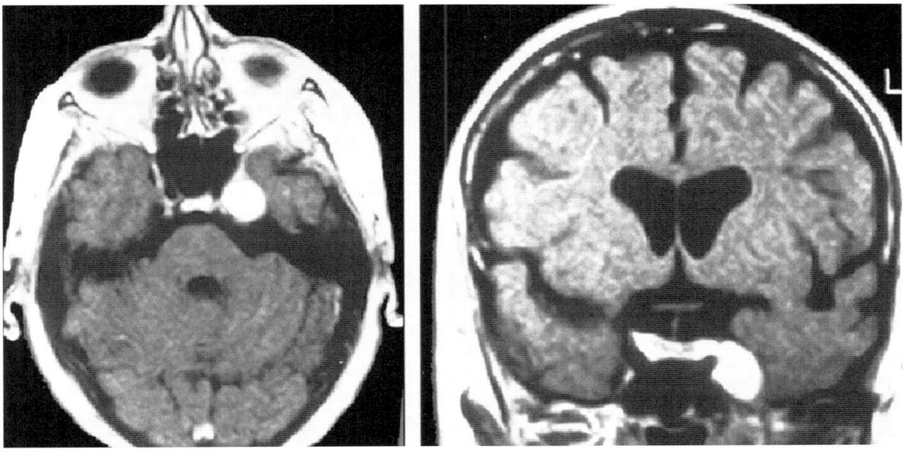

Figure 9–4 Trigeminal schwannoma. (A) Axial and (B) coronal infused T1-weighted magnetic resonance images demonstrating a smooth, circumscribed, enhancing mass in Meckel's cave. (With permission from Citow JS. Neuropathology and Neuroradiology: A Review. *New York, NY: Thieme Medical Publishers; 2001:105, Fig. 148.)*

A. Evaluation—evaluate for pheochromocytoma and renal cell carcinoma.

B. Treatment—surgical resection is carried out similar to AVM surgery by dissecting around the lesion and initially avoiding the veins.

C. Only 20% are associated with Von Hippel-Lindau Syndrome (CNS hemangioblastomas, retinal hemangiomas, renal cell carcinoma, pheochromocytoma, and cysts of the liver, pancreas, kidney).

XVII. CHORDOMA—usually located in the sacrum or clivus.

A. Treatment—wide en bloc surgical resection and XRT; prognosis usually poor

XVIII. EPIDERMOID AND DERMOID TUMORS

A. Treatment

1. Symptomatic—treat with surgical resection
2. Steroids—Mollaret's meningitis (inflammation by leakage of cholesterol crystals)

XIX. Lymphoma—metastatic lesions are usually meningeal, whereas primary intracranial lymphoma (usually in the immunocompromised) is usually located in the deep frontal or paraventricular region.

A. Evaluation

1. Hyperdense on CT, hyperintense on T1 MRI, and enhances strongly like a meningioma
2. Examination of lymph nodes, CXR, CT of the chest and abdomen, bone marrow biopsy, testicular ultrasound, and eye examination for uveitis

B. Treatment—tumors may disappear with steroids.

1. Biopsy
2. XRT—50 Gy 3/d fractions
3. Chemotherapy—intrathecal methotrexate in ventricular access device 12 mg 2/week × 6 with IV leukovorin rescue

C. Survival—3 months without treatment, 10 months with XRT

XX. Paragangliomas

A. Carotid body tumor

1. Signs/Symptoms—usually presents as a neck mass with cranial nerve X or XII palsy and ICA insufficiency
2. Evaluation—MRI and angiogram (ECA feeders and a splayed bifurcation). The tumors may release catecholamines and 5% are bilateral.
3. Treatment—resection (frequent cranial nerve X and XII injury 40%, CVA 10%, and death 10%) and XRT.

B. Glomus jugulare or tympanicu

1. Signs/Symptoms—usually presents with cranial nerve IX–XII palsies (jugulare) or cranial nerve VII and VIII palsy and bruit (tympanicum).
2. Evaluation
   a. Evaluate with otoscope—pulsatile red/blue mass behind eardrum
   b. Urine VMA—tumors may release catacholamines, seratonin, or histamine
   c. MRI and CT

3. Treatment—surgical resection (with preoperative embolization) and XRT.

   a. Histamine release at surgery may cause hypotension or bronchoconstriction; pretreat with 3 weeks of alpha-blockers and 3 days of beta-blockers.

XXI. Pediatric Tumors—juvenile pilocytic astrocytoma, medulloblastoma, brain stem glioma, and ependymoma. In children < 1 year, usually teratoma and glioblastoma (GBM).

XXII. Skull Tumors—epidermoid (scalloped margins); hemangioma (sunburst pattern); eosinophilic granuloma (punched-out lesion with clean margins, tender, associated with histiocytosis X); osteoma (sclerotic); and meningioma.

A. Treatment—en bloc resection if symptomatic

   1. Consider radiating a hemangioma if patient unable to tolerate surgery.

B. Tumors originating from various tissues—bone (osteoma and osteosarcoma), cartilage (chondroma and chondrosarcoma), fibrous (meningioma), marrow (multiple myeloma and histiocytoma), vessel (hemangioma), and other (fibrous dysplasia, Paget's disease, metastatic tumors).

XXIII. Metastases

A. Most frequent lesions—lung, breast, kidney, colon, and melanoma

B. Tumors that frequently hemorrhage—choriocarcinoma, renal cell carcinoma, and melanoma

C. Most common in children—neuroblastoma, rhabdomyosarcoma, and Wilms' tumor.

D. Drop mets—possible from medulloblastoma, ependymoma, pineal tumors, and GBM.

E. Evaluation—evaluate for primary tumor with CXR; CT of chest, abdomen, and pelvis; mammogram; bone scan

   1. Areas of diffuse ependymal enhancement are seen with leptomeningeal carcinomatosis or abscess.

F. Treatment
   1. Dilantin and steroids; possibly surgical resection and XRT
   2. Solitary met—excision and whole brain radiation therapy (WBRT) or stereotactic radiosurgery (SRS) if inaccessible.
   3. $\leq$ 3 mets—WBRT and SRS or surgery if accessible.
   4. $>$ 3 mets—WBRT.
   5. XRT—30 Gy over 2 weeks (sensitive tumors are small cell, germinoma, and lymphoma)
   6. Post-op XRT—questionable value

G. Survival—usually 6 months

XXIV. Neurofibromatosis Type 1 (NF-1)

A. Inclusion criteria are at least two of the following:
   1. Six café au lait spots
   2. Two neurofibromas
   3. One plexiform neurofibroma
   4. Axillary or inguinal freckling
   5. An osseous lesion (sphenoid dysplasia or thinning of long bones or cortex)
   6. An optic glioma
   7. Two Lisch nodules (iris hamartomas, only seen in NF-1)
   8. A relative with NF-1.

XXV. Neurofibromatosis Type 2

A. Associated tumors—bilateral vestibular schwannomas, meningiomas, astrocytomas, hamartomas, spinal ependymomas (spinal astrocytomas are more common in NF-1), and nerve root schwannomas

B. Inclusion criteria—bilateral vestibular schwannomas or a relative with NF-2 and one vestibular schwannoma, or two of the following:
   1. Neurofibroma, meningioma, glioma, schwannoma, or postcapsular cataract at a young age

C. Treatment—attempt to remove the vestibular schwannomas when small and try to preserve hearing in at least one ear. SRS may be of value.

XXVI. Tuberous Sclerosis

A. Signs/Symptoms—Classical triad is adenoma sebaceum (rashlike facial angiofibromas), mental retardation, and seizures.

B. Associated lesions

1. Cerebral hamartomas—tubers, frequently calcify, and usually don't enhance
2. Subependymal giant cell astrocytoma—enhances and is located near the foramen of Monro
3. Cardiac rhabdomyoma
4. Renal angiomyolipoma
5. Pancreatic adenoma
6. Retinal hamartoma
7. Cysts in the lung, liver, and spleen

C. Treatment—resect the astrocytoma if symptomatic (usually by hydrocephalus).

XXVII. Sturge-Weber Syndrome

A. Signs/Symptoms—ipsilateral V1 port-wine stain, cortical tram-track calcifications, and atrophy

B. Treatment—anticonvulsants and a skin-colored tatoo on the nevus flammeus

XXVIII. Spinal Tumors

A. Ependymoma—the most frequent tumor in the lower spinal cord

1. Treatment—surgical resection; use intraoperative nerve root monitoring (avoid paralytics).
2. Lesions of the cauda equina—section the upper filum first to prevent retraction (Fig. 9–5).

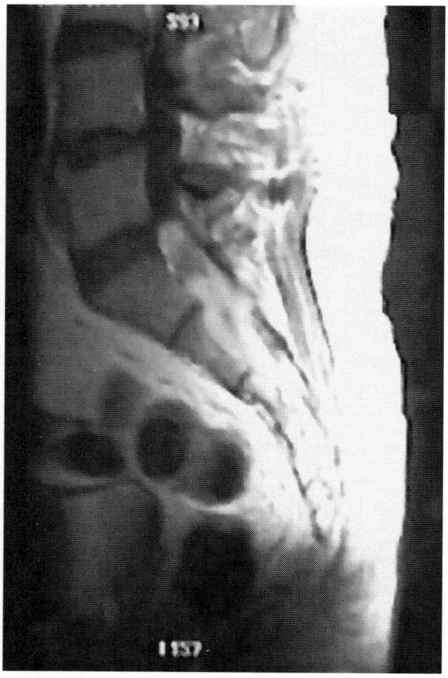

Figure 9–5 Myxopapillary ependymoma. Sagittal-infused, T1-weighted magnetic resonance image demonstrates enhancing nodular mass filling the distal spinal cord. (With permission from Citow JS. Neuropathology and Neuroradiology: A Review. *New York, NY: Thieme Medical Publishers; 2001:194, Fig. 266.)*

B. Astrocytoma—more common in children and in the upper spinal cord; usually low grade.

   1. Treatment—surgery (using SSEP monitoing) and XRT (only if not low grade) (Fig. 9–6)

C. Hemangioblastoma—usually cystic with a vascular mural nodule and located near the cord surface.

   1. Treatment—surgical resection

D. Vertebral hemangioma

   1. Ttreatment (only if symptomatic)—XRT, embolization, vertebroplasty, and surgical resection

E. Multiple myeloma (an isolated lesion is called a plasmacytoma)

   1. Evaluation—urinalysis (Bence Jones protein), CBC (anemia), blood serum electropheresis (IgG kappa chains), and skeletal bone survey
   2. Treatment—XRT and chemotherapy

F. Metastatic tumors

   1. Treatment

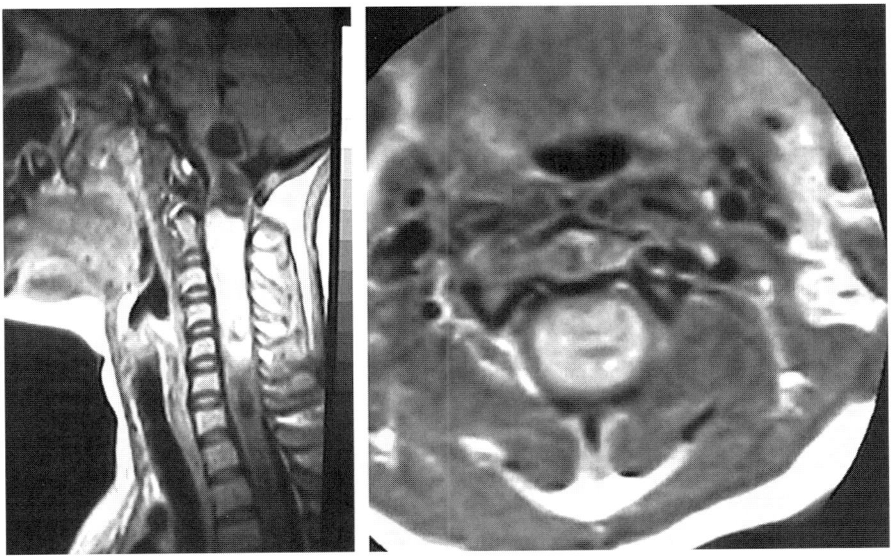

Figure 9–6 Intramedullary juvenile pilocytic astrocytoma. (A) Sagittal- and (B) axial-infused, T1-weighted magnetic resonance images demonstrate the enhancing tumor with the associated syrinx extending into the brain stem. (With permission from Citow JS. Neuropathology and Neuroradiology: A Review. *New York, NY: Thieme Medical Publishers; 2001:195, Fig. 268.)*

a. Surgery—indicated for unknown diagnosis, decompression, stabilization, and recurrence despite radiation

b. Steroids and XRT—30 Gy over 10 days, two levels above and below the tumor

XXIX. Radiation

A. Theory—x-rays and gamma rays deliver photons and particulate radiation to tumor cells to cause cell death and cessation of replication by freeing an electron to break bonds and produce free radicals to injure DNA. 1 Gy = 1 joule of energy absorbed/kg. 1 Gy = 100 rads. 1 cGy = 1 rad.

B. External beam radiation

1. Fractionation divides the dose to increase the therapeutic ratio (effect on tumor cells/normal cells).

2. Results depend on dose, time, and field. The body repairs sublethal damage.

3. Three Rs are redistribution (cells are most susceptible in the mitotic phase), repopulation (cell types change), and reoxygenation (cells are more susceptible with increased oxygen).
4. Delay XRT until 10 days postsurgery to allow initiation of healing.
5. Germinomas and lymphoma melt away but recur.

C. Radiation necrosis

1. Vascular endothelium and oligodendrogliomas are the most susceptible.
2. Usually occurs after 18 months
3. Radiation therapy lowers IQ 25 points (esp. doses > 40 Gy) and may injure the optic pathway and the pituitary/hypothalamic system, cause demyelination after methotrexate, and produce new tumors (GBM, meningioma, or osteosarcoma).
4. Evaluation—MR-spectroscopy or PET scan (increased glucose use in tumors decreases with necrosis).
5. Treatment
   a. Only resect necrosis if there is mass effect.
   b. Prevent necrosis by keeping the radiation dose < 60 Gy over 6 weeks; in the spinal cord avoid doses > 0.2 Gy/d.

D. Stereotactic radiosurgery

1. General
   a. Best for AVMs or tumors < 3 cm and inaccessible
   b. 2-year latency with AVM therapy before the hemorrhage risk decreases
   c. Use multiple ports with a steep gradient drop-off to decrease surrounding brain injury.
2. Linear accelerator (LINAC)
   a. Photon beam is made by electron acceleration (x-ray).
   b. More flexible and less expensive than gamma knife with nonspherical lesions
   c. Results—similar to gamma knife
   d. Modification of target—produced by changing arc paths and collimator size

3. Gamma knife
   a. Photon beam is made by natural radioactive decay (gamma ray)
   b. Narrower distribution of energy produces slightly better spatial accuracy than LINAC, but this is less than the error in target margins (LINAC has 1 mm error).
   c. Uses different-sized collimators and exposure times and > 1 isocenter.
   d. Target modification—performed by plugging collimators passing radiation through sensitive areas
4. Fractionated stereotactic radiosurgery (radiotherapy)
   a. Reoxygenation helps kill more cells.
   b. Fractionation hits late responders and multiple cell cycles.
   c. Hypofractionation—1 fraction/d $\times$ 1 week; best for slow-growing benign tumors (meningioma, schwannoma, and AVM)
5. Planning
   a. Use five arcs 100 degrees each to keep the drop-off optimal.
   b. Tissue 2.5 mm away will be injured.
   c. CT localizes better than MRI due to magnetic artifact, but accuracy can't be < 0.6 mm due to pixel size (MRI shift is 2 mm).
   d. Multiple isocenters help conform to an irregular shape.
6. Specific lesions
   a. AVM—perform 30 days after embolization (avoid radiopaque dye). Use 15 Gy to the periphery of the lesion. Obliteration rate is 50% at 1 year and 86% at 2 years.
   b. Schwannoma—use 14 Gy at 80% isodense line. 40% shrink and 40% stop growing.
   c. Metastatic tumors—use 15 Gy at the center at 80% isodense curve.
7. Complications—headache, emesis, seizures (premedicate with Decadron 10 mg and phenobarbital 90 mg), radiation necrosis 3%, symptomatic white matter changes 20%, vascular changes 5%, and cranial nerve dysfunction 1%.

XXX. Surgical Approaches

A. Temporal lobe lesions

1. Treatment

a. Safe to remove 5 cm of the dominant side and 7 cm of nondominant side (overresection to the optic radiations causes a visual field cut)

b. Start removal of the temporal lobe from the tip and work posteriorly.

c. Be careful with the uncus (near the tentorium and 3rd nerve) and MCA branches in the sylvian fissure (stay in a subpial plane).

d. Enter through the middle temporal gyrus and spare the superior temporal gyrus.

e. Consider lateral or supine patient position.

f. Skin incision may be horseshoe anterior and posterior to the ear, question mark extending posterior to the ear, or linear (for anterior lesions) (Fig. 9–7).

B. Lateral ventricle atrium (trigone)—patient in lateral position; enter through the middle temporal gyrus, lateral temporoparietal cortex, or the superior parieto-occipital region

C. Frontal horn of lateral ventricle—patient in supine position; enter through the middle frontal gyrus

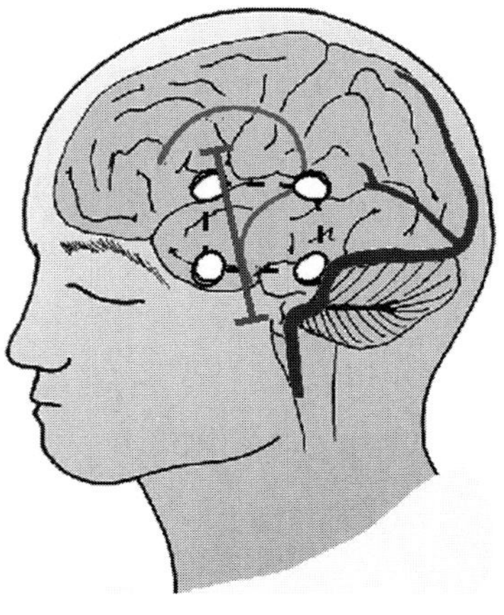

Figure 9–7 Temporal lobe exposure.

D. Body of lateral ventricle—patient in supine position; transcallosal approach

E. Third ventricle—patient in supine position; transcallosal approach (less seizure risk than with transcortical approach).

1. Author prefers a linear incision to a horseshoe incision in this and most procedures.
2. Be careful with superior sagittal sinus retraction, the surrounding veins, and the fornix.
3. Incise only 2.5 cm of the anterior corpus callosum.
4. Disconnection syndrome more likely with posterior incision through the splenium.
5. Fenestrate the lateral ventricle and then proceed into the third ventricle via an interforniceal approach or extend the foramen of Monro posteriorly by opening the choroidal fissure or anteriorly through fornix (some say one fornix can be removed with little memory deficit).
6. Prepare both sides of the head in case interhemispheric veins are prohibitive (Figs. 9–8, 9–9).

F. Anterior fossa skull base—for olfactory groove meningiomas, etc.

1. Patient in supine position
2. Bicoronal incision is made connecting the two zygomatic arches.
3. The scalp flap should be dissected forward above the pericranium to provide a flap for closure.
4. Dissection over the temporalis muscles should be in the interfascial plane or below the fascia when the fat pads are reached to avoid injuring the frontalis branch of the facial nerve.
5. Burr holes are placed at the keyholes and around the anterior superior sagittal sinus; bone flap is turned.
6. Anterior $\frac{1}{3}$ of the sinus may usually be sacrificed when needed.
7. Frontal sinus should be cranialized by removing the posterior wall and removing the mucosa.
8. Frontal osteum should be plugged with muscle.
9. Blood supply is usually under the lesion; try to ligate as early as possible.

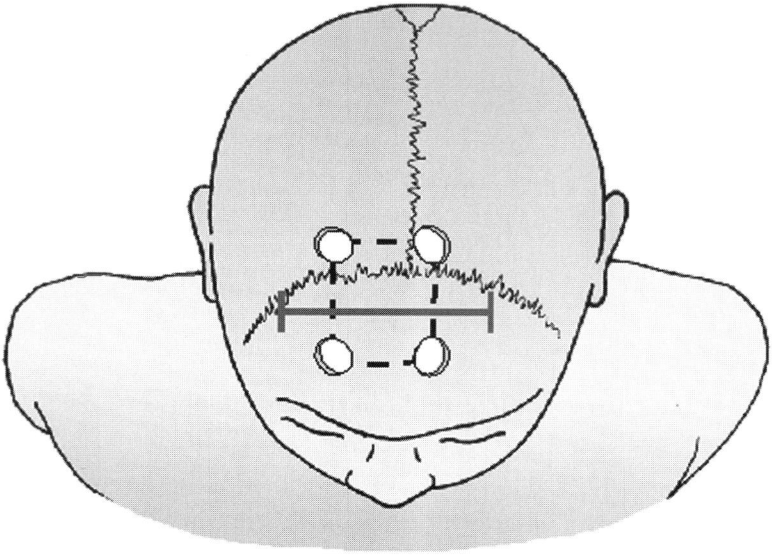

Figure 9–8 *Transcallosal exposure.*

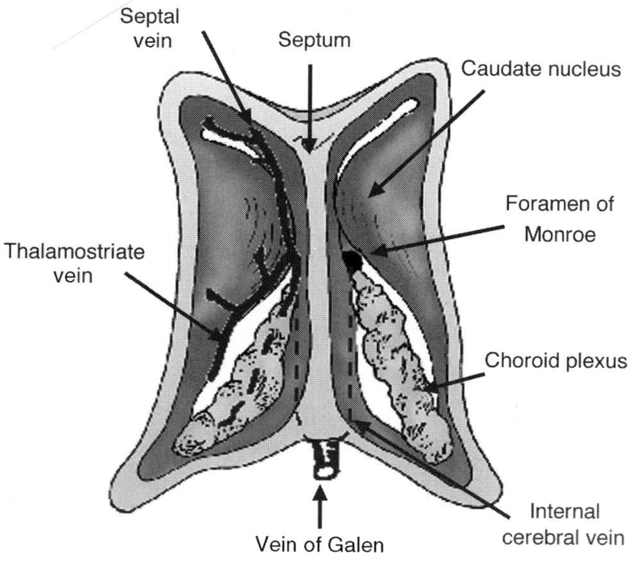

Figure 9–9 *View inside the lateral ventricles.*

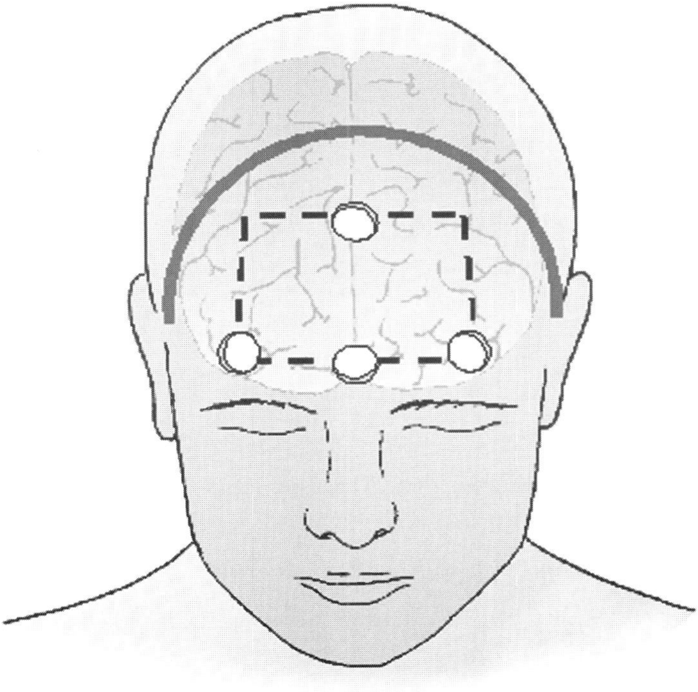

Figure 9–10 Bicoronal craniotomy incision.

10. At closure, the pericranial flap should be placed over the base of the anterior fossa and sutured to the planum sphenoidalum dura.
11. Outer dura should then be closed in a water-tight fashion.
12. CSF leak should be treated with a lumbar drain and intermittent skull x-rays to watch for pneumocephalus.
13. Complications—injury to cranial nerves I (almost always) and II, brain injury (cognitive impairment and seizures), anterior cerebral artery injury, and infection (Fig. 9–10).

G. Transpetrosal approach—used to expose anterior or lateral lesions from the midbrain to the lower pons (i.e., cavernous malformation, clivus chordoma, and petroclival meningioma) (Fig. 9–11).

1. Patient postioned with falx parallel to floor (usually lateral).
2. Horseshoe incision is fashioned from the base of the mastoid, around the pinna, to the zygoma.
3. Zygoma, mastoid, and external auditory canal are identified.

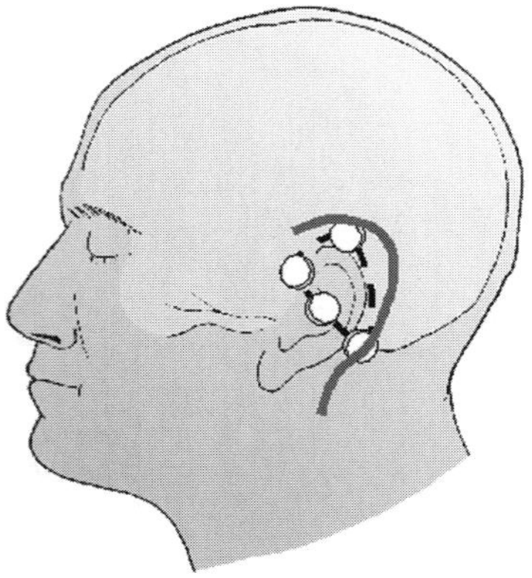

Figure 9–11 *Transpetrosal craniotomy.*

4. Locate the asterion (junction of the parietomastoid, occipitomastoid, and lambdoid sutures) that overlies the junction of the transverse and sigmoid sinuses.
5. Transverse sinus is usually under the superior nuchal line.
6. Burr holes are placed on both sides of the transverse and sigmoid sinuses.
7. Do not dissect across the sinus with a Penfield #3; instead use a kerasin punch.
8. Remove the boomerang-shaped bone flap.
9. Drill off the mastoid bone to expose the semicirclar canals and the superior petrosal sinus (in the dural at the junction of the tentorium, middle, and posterior fossa).
10. Maximize bony removal to minimize brain retraction.
11. Open the presigmoid dura and divide the superior petrosal sinus.
12. Locate the trochlear nerve under the tentorium.
13. Operative window is between cranial nerves V/VII and VII/IX.
14. The exposure will not reach lesions below the jugular foramen.
15. Close with a fat graft, fibrin glue, and a lumbar drain to prevent CSF leak (as high as 20%).
16. Complications—injury to the cranial nerves, hearing loss by damage to the semicircular canals with loss of endolymph (be sure to obtain a pre-op contralateral audiogram), and sinus injury.

H. Anterior foramen magnum lesions—consider transoral approach (see rheumatoid arthritis section), far lateral (transcondylar), or posterior approaches.

I. Far lateral (transcondylar) approach—for lesions involving the lower $\frac{1}{3}$ of clivus to the upper cervical spine (contralateral vertebrobasilar junction aneurysm).

1. Patient is positioned prone with the involved side rotated 30 degrees up.
2. Incision is made over the spinous processes of C1–3 and curved laterally over the mastoid bone.
3. Vertebral artery is identified at the superior C1 transverse arch as it pierces the dura to move up the foramen magnum.
4. Greater occipital nerve may be identified and followed down to the C2 nerve root.
5. C1 hemilaminectomy is performed and the foramen magnum is opened.
6. Lateral mass of C1 and posteromedial occipital condyle are drilled off to the hypoglossal canal (if more is removed, an occipitocervical fusion is needed).
7. Vertebral artery is mobilized from the C2 arch to the foramen magnum and retracted medially (Fig. 9–12).

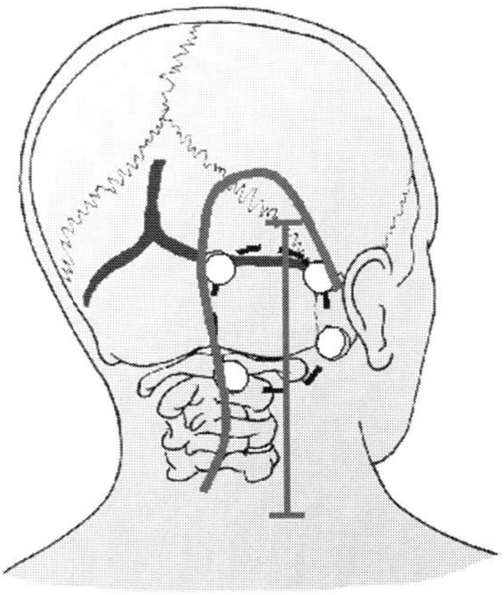

Figure 9–12 Far-lateral (transcondylar) incision.

J. Perforate methylmethacrylate if used as a skull replacement to decrease the fluid accumulation under the bone flap.

K. Intraoperative brain swelling—consider edema, blood clot, hydrocephalus, internal jugular vein occlusion, or hypercapnea.

   1. Evaluation—intraoperative ultrasound

   2. Treatment—mannitol, Lasix, hyperventilation, and ventricular drainage

      a. Always consider placement of an occipital Frazier burr hole with posterior fossa surgery.

CHAPTER 10

Cerebrovascular Disease

I. Stroke

A. Transient ischemic attack (TIA)—deficit lasts < 24 hours.

B. Reversible ischemic neurological deficit (RIND)—deficit lasts < 1 week.

C. Cerebrovascular accident (CVA)—stroke, deficit lasts > 1 week.

D. Amaurosis fugax—transient monocular blindness usually due to a small fibrin embolus.

E. CVA risk after an ocular TIA—17% in 2 years

F. CVA risk after a hemispheric TIA—43% in 2 years (usually within 3 months)

G. CVA etiologies

1. 60% from atherosclerosis—possibly from an embolic plaque or ischemia, usually 50% stenosis is necessary to be symptomatic
2. 20% lacunar—small-vessel lipohyalinosis
3. 15% from cardiac embolism
4. 15% of CVAs are hemorrhage; 85% are dry.

H. Cerebral autoregulation

1. Occurs with cerebral perfusion pressure (CPP) 50–150 mmHg to keep cerebral blood flow (CBF) normal (around 55 mL/100g of brain tissue/min)
2. Ischemic penumbra—area where cells receive a CBF of 18–23 mm Hg, enough to survive but not enough to be functional (these cells may survive to restore function over time)

I. CVA symptoms

1. Carotid circulation—unilateral motor, sensory, visual, or speech deficit
2. Vertebral circulation—bilateral motor, sensory, or visual deficits, or syncope

J. Evaluation

1. History—tobacco use, elevated cholesterol, hypertension, diabetes, angina, and claudication
2. Physical Evaluation—funduscopy, assessment of superficial temporal artery (STA) pulses, bruits
3. Lavoratory Evaluation—CBC, platelets, PT/PTT, electrolytes, ABG, RPR (syphilis), ESR, EKG, and 24-hour cardiac monitor
4. Radiologic Evaluation
   a. CT
      i. Initially may be normal or with edema
      ii. After one week shows gyral ribbon enhancement
      iii. Many weeks later reveals atrophy
   b. Carotid duplex—combines color flow Doppler and β-mode ultrasound.
      i. Doppler effect—change in sound pitch as sound waves hit a moving target; the frequency decreases as it leaves and increases as it approaches.
   c. Carotid and cerebral MRA or angiogram—may demonstrate a string sign or occluded vessels as well as luxury perfusion (increased CBF adjacent to a CVA due to impaired autoregulation from the acidosis). Don't operate if a tandem cerebral lesion is more stenotic than the carotid lesion.

K. Thrombolytic therapy

1. Reverse t-PA use does not change the deficit at 24 hours but improves it at 3 months; 30% of patients are more likely to have little or no deficit.
2. Must be administered within 3 hours of symptoms
3. Exclusion criteria—CT with edema or hemorrhage, SBP > 185 mm Hg, seizures, anticoagulants, surgery within 14 days, CVA within 3 months, or glucose > 400

4. Increased risk of intraparenchymal hemorrhage 6.4% from 0.6%, though the mortality stays at 20%
5. Dose—0.09 mg/kg IV over 1 minute and then 0.81 mg/kg over 60 minutes
6. Reverse t-PA for surgery—Amicar 5 g IV (acts in 15 minutes), cryoprecipitate, and FFP

L. CVA treatment
1. IV fluid without dextrose
2. Aspirin (ASA)—325 mg PO qd
3. Maintain SBP < 180 mm Hg (but > 130 mm Hg)
4. The risk of another CVA is 1%/week with or without heparin (not recommended).
5. Coumadin—use only for antiphospholipid antibody, atrial fibrillation, or vertebral insufficiency.
6. Craniectomy—may be used for cerebellar or right middle cerebral artery CVAs with excessive mass effect.
7. Avoid hyperthermia and hyperglycemia; they make the neurons more vulnerable to ischemia.

M. Best medical management
1. Start with ASA (325 mg qd) or Ticlid to produce a 30% decrease in CVA rate after a TIA.
2. Ticlid and Plavix may lower the WBC count.
3. Control hypertension, diabetes, cholesterol, and tobacco use.
4. Anticoagulation—for atrial fibrillation or vertebrobasilar symptoms.
5. Heparin (converted to Coumadin)—if there is $> 95\%$ stenosis

N. Surgical management
1. Degree of stenosis—as per the NASCET study $(1 - a/b) \times 100$ is the percent stenosis (Figs. 10–1, 10–2).
2. Asymptomatic carotid atherosclerosis study (ACAS)
   a. If there is $> 60\%$ stenosis, surgery decreases the CVA rate only if the complication rate is $< 3\%$.

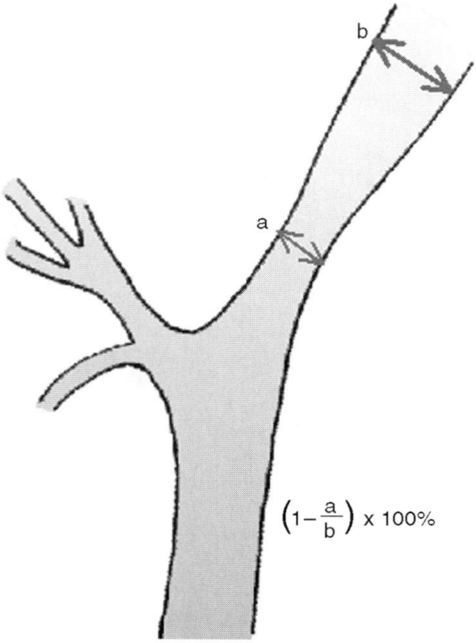

Figure 10–1 *Carotid stenosis diagram.*

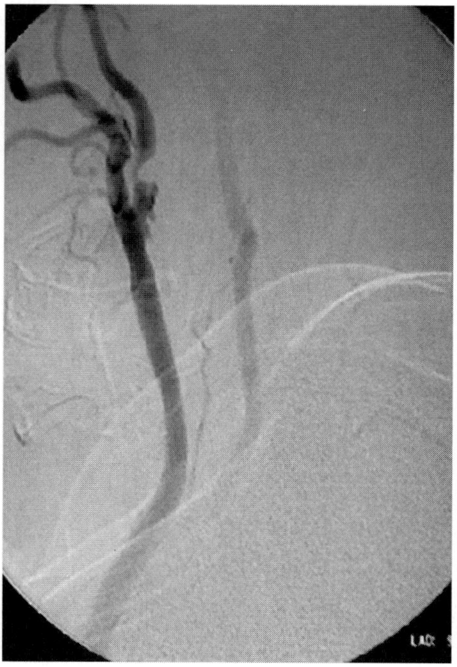

Figure 10–2 *Carotid artery stenosis. Angiogram demonstrates proximal internal carotid artery plaque. (With permission from Citow JS.* Neuropathology and Neuroradiology: A Review. *New York, NY: Thieme Medical Publishers; 2001:149, Fig. 194.)*

b. 5-year CVA rate decreased 66% in males and 17% in females (however, there was no decrease in major CVA rate or death)

c. 5-year CVA rate without surgery was 11% and with surgery was 5%.

3. NASCET

a. In the presence of a hemispheric or retinal TIA and stenosis > 70%, surgery decreases the CVA rate 17% and the death rate 7% over 1.5 years.

b. 2-year CVA rate is 40% without ASA, 26% with ASA, and 9% with ASA and carotid endarterectomy (CEA).

c. There is a 1%/month risk of CVA while waiting for surgery.

4. Recommendations

a. Asymptomatic carotid stenosis—only operate if > 60% stenosis

b. Symptomatic carotid stenosis—operate if > 50% stenosis

5. Carotid endarterectomy

a. Perform 2–6 weeks after CVA and perform another ultrasound immediately before surgery to detect any changes.

b. Sundt morbidity and mortality scale—risk factors are myocardial infarction, hypertension, COPD, CVA within 7 days, carotid siphon stenosis, and contralateral stenosis.

c. Preoperative ASA 325 mg qd × 5 days and resume post-op at 48 hours.

i. Ticlid reverses in 2 hours with methylprednisolone.

ii. Change over to ASA before surgery.

d. Selective shunting—based on EEG changes (1–4% require a shunt).

i. EEG changes—usually caused by a shower of cholesterol plaques, not blood clots.

ii. Treatment—heparin 5000 U, thiopental 3 mg/kg, raise the SBP to 170 mm Hg, shunt, and consider angiography with possible urokinase or embolectomy

e. Patch implantation—if small vessel, long plaque, or repeat surgery

f. Exposure
   i. Make the skin incision over the medial border of the sternocleidomastoid (SCM).
   ii. Watch for the greater auricular nerve over the SCM (section causes numbness in the jaw and ear).
   iii. Expose the digastric muscle proximally and omohyoid muscle distally.
   iv. Divide the common facial vein.
   v. Follow the descendent hypoglossi to cranial nerve XII.
   vi. Place loops around the common carotid artery (CCA), internal carotid artery (ICA), external carotid artery (ECA), and superior thyroid artery (Fig. 10–3).
g. Clamping
   i. Bolus with heparin 70 U/kg 5 minutes before clamping.
   ii. Clamp first the ICA, the CCA, the superior thyroid artery, and then the ECA (aneurysm clips on all but a vascular clamp on the CCA).
   iii. After the endarterectomy, suture the vessel closed with 5.0 Proline.
   iv. Unclamp first the ECA and flush the CCA and ICA.
   v. Open the CCA and finally the ICA.

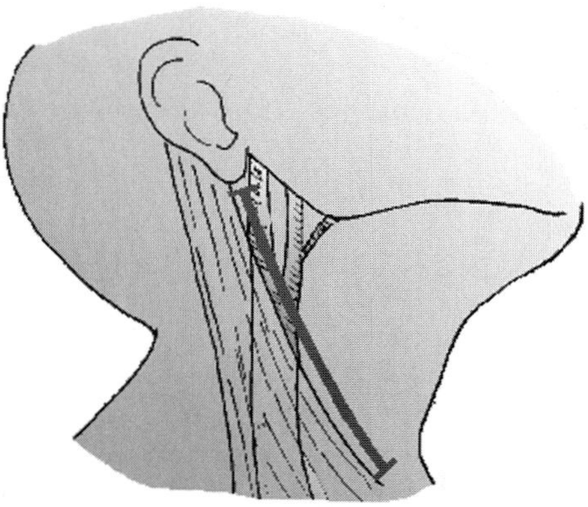

Figure 10–3 Carotid endarterectomy incision.

h. Emergent CEA
   i. Only used if there is a sudden deficit with a lost bruit in the presence of known stenosis, during angiography, or after CEA
   ii. Don't operate on a totally occluded carotid artery after 2 hours if there is a fixed deficit.
   iii. There is a 3%/year CVA risk from stump embolism with complete occlusion.
i. Complications
   i. Injuries to cranial nerve XII—near the facial vein
   ii. Injuries to recurrent laryngeal nerve—near the trachea; keep the medial retractor at the platysma
   iii. Injuries to superior laryngeal nerve—dysphasia; avoid by starting dissection lateral to the carotid artery
   iv. Reactive cerebral hyperemia
   v. Recurrence—stenosis recurs in 20% of patients over 10 years.

6. Post-op evaluation
   1. Look for pronator drift, dysphasia, papillary reactivity, STA pulses (to find ECA or CCA occlusion), tongue deviation, hoarseness, and hematoma with dysphagia or tracheal deviation.
   2. Beware of vessel leak, pseudoaneurysm, TIA/CVA, cerebral hemorrhage, or seizure.
   3. Cranial nerve injuries
      a. X—vocal cord paralysis or hoarseness
      b. XII—tongue deviation
      c. VII—lip depressor weakness from mandibular branch
   4. Possible hypertension from loss of baroreceptor reflex
   5. Post-op TIA—evaluate with CT and angiogram
   6. Fixed post-op CVA
      a. Return to OR and reopen the vessel (clamp the CCA and ECA, open the ICA to see backflow, try to insert a Fogerty #4 catheter to remove the clot).
      b. Use aggressive IV fluids to increase the SBP to 180 mmHg, increase O_2, and use pressors if needed.

c. A neck hematoma may need to be removed to enable intubation (try once, don't paralyze the patient, open the neck in the OR).

d. Consider performing a CT if there is a nonlocalizing deficit.

7. Angioplasty

a. Currently used in the elderly, infirm, those with recurrent stenosis, post-XRT stenosis, or evolving CVA despite thrombolytics

b. Risk of embolism and subintimal dissection

c. Stent may be placed after angioplasty

O. CVA outcome—25% mortality, 25% disabled, 50% return home

P. CVA from cardiac embolism

1. Accounts for $\frac{1}{6}$ of CVAs.

2. 2% of MIs develop a CVA within 2 weeks.

3. Without anticoagulation—risk of CVA with atrial fibrillation is 4.5%/year and with a bioprosthetic heart valve is 3%/year

4. With anticoagulation—risk of CVA with a mechanical mitral valve is 3%/year and a mechanical aortic valve is 1.5%/year

5. Evaluation

a. Rule out a paradoxical embolism from a patent foramen ovale in young patients that suffer a CVA.

b. Rule out cerebrovascular disease and a source for an embolism (echocardiogram and EKG).

c. There is frequent hemorrhagic transformation at 48 hours.

6. Treatment

a. No proven benefit with early anticoagulation—12% CVA risk in 2 weeks vs. risk of hemorrhagic transformation

b. Perform CT at 2 days—if no clot, use heparin and Coumadin together for 3 days until the INR is 2–3.

c. Coumadin use with atrial fibrillation decreases the CVA risk 75% vs 40% with ASA.

Q. Young CVA patients—search for deficiencies of protein C and S and antithrombin III, and the presence of factor 5 leiden, antiphospholipid antibody, systemic lupus erythromatosis (SLE), syphilis, tuberculosis, diabetes, hypertension, tobacco use, and increased cholesterol.

R. Lacunar CVA—from small-vessel disease by lipohyalinosis of MCA branches.

1. Signs/Symptoms
   a. No cortical symptoms
   b. Most common manifestation is pure sensory loss.
   c. Less common syndromes are pure motor hemiparesis or ataxic hemiparesis.
2. Treatment—carotid endarterectomy does not help.

S. Lateral medullary syndrome (Wallenberg's syndrome)

1. Cause—vertebral or PICA occlusion
2. Signs/Symptoms—ipsilateral vertigo (VIII), facial numbness (V), dysphagia (IX,X), Horner's syndrome, cerebellar ataxia, loss of light touch in the ipsilateral body (posterior columns), and contralateral loss of pain/temperature (spinothalamic tract).

T. Vertebrobasilar insufficiency

1. Cause—usually subclavian steal or vessel stenosis
2. Signs/Symptoms
   a. 5 Ds—diplopia, dysarthria, defect visual, dizzy, drop attack
   b. Bilateral motor, sensory, or visual symptoms.
3. Treatment—decrease risk factors, medications (Coumadin or ASA), and surgery (endarterectomy, VA–ICA transposition, or bypass)

U. Internal carotid artery dissection

1. Signs/Symptoms—pain, oculosympathetic Horner's syndrome (sweat fibers travel with the ECA), cranial nerve XII deficit, TIA (due to embolism or occlusion), and subarachnoid hemorrhage (SAH).
2. Evaluation
   a. Angiogram with string sign or double lumen (dissection occurs 2 cm distal to the CCA bifurcation)

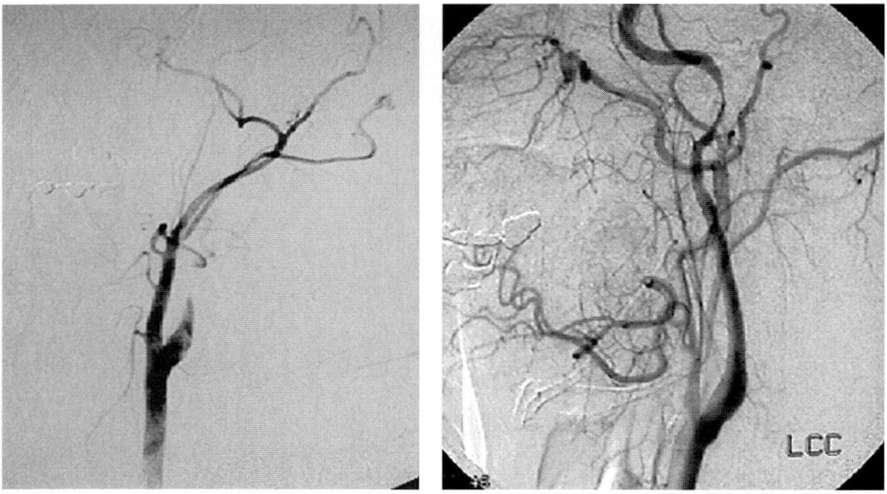

Figure 10–4 *Carotid artery dissection. (A) Angiograms demonstrate cervical internal carotid artery (ICA) and (B) petrous ICA tapered narrowings. (With permission from Citow JS.* Neuropathology and Neuroradiology: A Review. *New York, NY: Thieme Medical Publishers; 2001:155, Fig. 200.)*

b. Associated with cystic medial necrosis, fibromuscular dysplasia, Ehlers-Danlos syndrome, Marfan's syndrome, and syphilis (Fig. 10–4A,B)

3. Treatment

a. Heparin 2 weeks followed by Coumadin 12 weeks

b. If symptoms progress, consider direct surgical repair, ligation, stenting, or bypass (STA–MCA or high flow).

c. If there is a large CVA or a complete deficit, use ASA and hold the Coumadin for 2 weeks.

V. Vertebral dissection—usually occurs between C1 and 2 or at C6 (where the artery enters the foramen transversarium).

1. Signs/Symptoms

a. Neck pain, CVA (lateral medullary syndrome), or subarachnoid hemorrhage.

b. Extradural lesions usually present with stroke from embolism or vessel occlusion, whereas intradural lesions present with SAH.

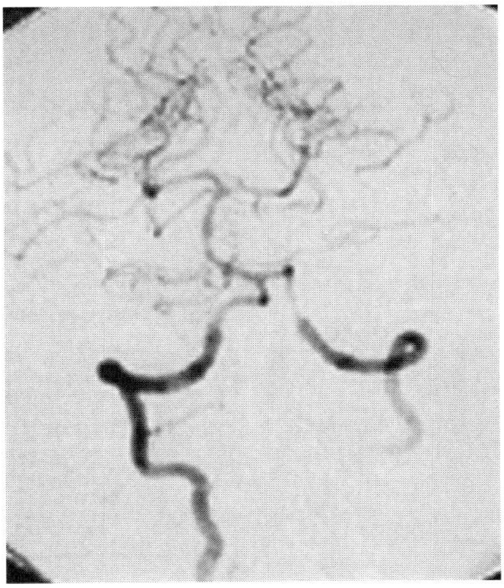

Figure 10–5 Vertebral artery dissection. Angiogram demonstrates left distal vertebral artery narrowing. (With permission from Citow JS. Neuropathology and Neuroradiology: A Review. *New York, NY: Thieme Medical Publishers; 2001:156, Fig. 201.)*

2. Treatment—heparin and Coumadin for 6 months (don't anticoagulate in the presence of a large CVA or SAH) or trap the vessel proximal to PICA if possible (open procedure or endovascular with a balloon) (Fig. 10–5)

W. Venous sinus thrombosis

1. Causes—related to infection, dehydration, pregnancy, OCPs, and deficiency of proteins C, S, antithrombin III, and factor 5 leiden.
2. Evaluation—CT and MRV.
3. Treatment
   a. Address the primary disorder, increase hydration, and use heparin and Coumadin.
   b. If symptoms are increasing, use t-PA or urokinase to lyse the clot.
   c. Consider endovascular therapy from the femoral vein to the superior sagittal sinus with 25 mg t-PA as a 2 mg bolus at each end of the sinus; advance the catheter to the anterior sinus and infuse 1 mg/min × 19 min.
   e. Anticoagulation is safe in the presence of scattered punctate hemorrhages from venous occlusive disease.

X. Moyamoya disease—bilateral distal ICA occlusion with rete mirabile (transdural ECA anastamoses causing a puff-of-smoke appearance).

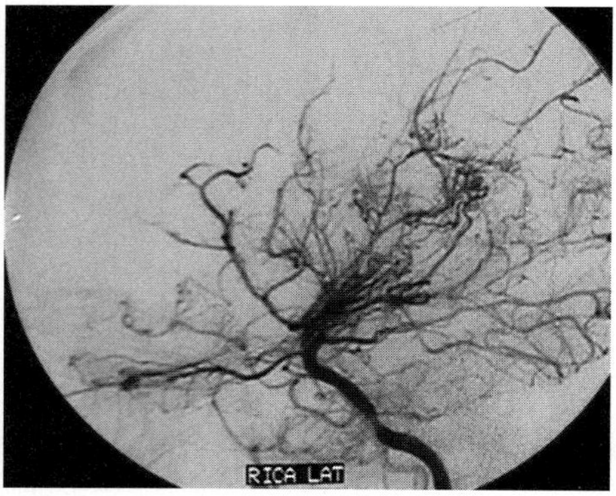

Figure 10–6 Moyamoya disease. Angiogram demonstrates distal internal carotid artery occlusion with prominent leptomeningeal collaterals ("puff of smoke"). (With permission from Citow JS. Neuropathology and Neuroradiology: A Review. *New York, NY: Thieme Medical Publishers; 2001:154, Fig. 199.)*

1. Signs/Symptoms—in children are from CVA; in adults are from hemorrhage
2. Evaluation—MRI and angiogram (there are frequently aneurysms) (Fig. 10–6)
3. Treatment
   a. Medical therapy is of unknown benefit.
   b. Surgical treatment—STA–MCA bypass, encephalomyosynangiosis (temporal muscle to brain), encephaloduroarteriosynangiosis (STA branches placed inside a dural opening), or an omental flap.
   c. Encephaloduralsynangiosis
      i. Identify the STA and middle meningeal artery branches on the angiogram.
      ii. Palpate the STA and locate with a Doppler; incise around it with 15-blade knife.
      iii. Make two burr holes and connect with a craniotomy.
      iv. Open the dura where avascular and sew the STA adventitia to the pia with 10.0 Proline.
      v. Lay down the dura and bone.
      vi. Make a few more burr holes.

II. Intraparenchymal Hemorrhage

A. Hypertensive hemorrhage—most common locations are putamen 60%, thalamus 20%, pons 10%, and cerebellum 5% (near the dentate nucleus).

1. Signs/Symptoms
    a. Headache, weakness, and dysphasia
    b. Pontine hemorrhages may produce pinpoint pupils and "locked-in syndrome."
    c. Cerebellar hemorrhages present with contralateral eye deviation, focal weakness but not hemiplegia, and a rapid loss of consciousness.
    d. Most patients have a history of hypertension and usually present to the ER with an SBP over 180 mmHg.
2. Treatment
    a. Lower the blood pressure 30% with Nipride (overaggressive lowering to a "normal range" may lead to hypoperfusion CVA).
    b. Anticonvulsants—usually not needed
    c. Re-hemorrhage—relatively rare
    d. Ventricular extension in up to 50% of cases—may require external ventricular drainage
    e. Surgery—not proven to improve functional outcome with putamen or thalamic clots, though mortality may be decreased.
    f. Surgical evacuation—for cerebellar clots > 4 cm or with hydrocephalus
    g. Functional outcome—best with volumes 10–30 mL

B. Amyloid angiopathy
1. Usually occurs in older patients
2. Most common cause of lobar hemorrhage in normotensive elderly patients.
3. Clot typically extends from the centrum semiovale to the subarachnoid space.
4. Cause of the hemorrhage is replacement of the contractile elements in the media of the arteries and arterioles of the leptomeningeal and superficial cortical vessels with noncontractile amyloid that is yellow-green with dichromism (birefringence) when stained with Congo red dye and viewed under polarized light.

C. "Iatrogenic"

1. Hemorrhage rate in CVA patients treated with t-PA is 6%; in those with MI treated with t-PA it is 2%.

2. Risk of cerebral hemorrhage with Coumadin therapy for atrial fibrillation is 0.3%/year.

3. Delay for 1 week anticoagulation after intraparenchymal hemorrhage in patients with mechanical heart valves.

D. Evaluation—consider evaluation of an intraparenchymal hemorrhage with an angiogram (to rule out vascular lesions) in patients < 45 years and with no history of hypertension.

E. Multiple intraparenchymal hemorrhages in young patients

1. Causes—trauma, drug abuse (cocaine), vasculitis systemic lupus erythematosis, Wegener's granulomatosis, polyarteritis nodosa, infection, or coagulopathy

F. Multiple intraparenchymal hemorrhage in older patients

1. Causes—amyloid angiopathy, embolic CVA, vasculitis, syphilis, or metastatic tumor

III. Cerebral Aneurysms

A. Causes of spontaneous subarachnoid hemorrhage

1. Aneurysm 80% and vascular malformation 10%

2. By far, the most common cause of subarachnoid hemorrhage overall is trauma.

B. Conditions associated with aneurysms—hypertension, atherosclerosis, fibromuscular dysplasia (FMD), polycystic kidney disease, Ehlers-Danlos syndrome, and Marfan's syndrome.

C. Rupture rate—according to the recent NEJM study, the rupture rate of unruptured aneurysms < 10 mm is 0.05%/y and > 10 mm is 1%/year. However, these numbers may be misleading because the most common rupture size is 6–9 mm.

1. Morbidity and mortality per rupture—5% in patients < 30 years and 30% in patients > 60 years

2. The surgical mortality/morbidity for clipping is around 5%.

3. It is probably worthwhile to scan first-degree relatives of aneurysm patients with an MRA given that 20% of patients have a family member with at least one.

D. Re-rupture rate of ruptured aneurysms

1. 4% in 24 hours, 20% in 2 weeks, 50% in 6 months, and then 3%/y

2. Re-rupture rate for a "dog-ear" incompletely clipped aneurysm is 0.4%/y

E. Outcome—40% mortality, 30% disabled, 30% normal, 10% die at home

F. Hunt and Hess grade

0—unruptured aneurysm

1—asymptomatic or mild headache and slight nuchal rigidity

1a—no acute meningeal/brain reaction, but with fixed neuro deficit

2—cranial nerve palsy, moderate to severe headache, nuchal rigidity

3—mild focal deficit, lethargy or confusion

4—stupor, moderate to severe hemiparesis, early decerebrate

5—deep coma, decerebrate posturing, moribund appearance.

Add one grade for serious systemic disease (HTN, DM, etc.) or severe vasospasm on angiogram.

G. Evaluation

1. History—sudden onset of worst headache in life

2. CT, LP (if CT negative)

3. Four-vessel angiogram—20% are multiple

4. MRI/MRA—only if angiogram equivocal

5. CT angiography—gaining popularity

6. Ocular examination—may reveal subhyaloid preretinal, retinal, or vitreous hemorrhage (Terson's syndrome, due to elevated ICP and venous pressure, usually resolves in 6 months, may need vitrectomy).

7. Alcock test—vertebral angiogram with carotid compression to test competency of the circle of Willis.

8. Determine aneurysm size—compare to the diameter of the ICA (6 mm) and MCA (4 mm).

H. Fisher grade (for vasospasm, per CT)

1—no subarachnoid blood

2—diffuse blood or vertical layers < 1 mm thick

3—localized clot and/or vertical layer ≥ 1 mm thick

4—intracerebral or intraventricular clot with diffuse or no subarachnoid hemorrhage

Grades 1,2, and 4 usually do not develop vasospasm.

Grade 3 patients frequently develop vasospasm.

I. Treatments

1. Nipride to keep SBP 120–130 mm Hg to prevent re-hemorrhage prior to surgery.
2. Studies suggest that surgery should be performed the same day or the following morning.
3. Gold standard treatment—surgical clipping
4. Endovascular coiling
   a. Growing in popularity, but as of now, > 20% need re-treatment and the morbidity/mortality is > 5%
   b. Most useful for straight-shot aneurysms with difficult exposure (basilar apex, basilar trunk, and superior hypophyseal), multiple aneurysms, and aneurysms with a dome:neck ratio > 1.
5. Muslin wrapping—not proven to be of benefit
6. Trapping with or without bypass may be needed for unclippable aneurysms.
7. During surgery
   a. Achieve brain relaxation with mannitol (1 g/kg bolus), Lasix, hyperventilation, and ventricular drainage (or lumbar drainage).
   b. Maintain normotension (but use mild hypertension during temporary clipping) and mild hypothermia (to 32–34°C with passive drift).
8. Temporary clipping time > 5 minutes—use Pentothal (4 mg/kg bolus and 2 mg/kg/h titrated to burst suppression if available), propofol (170 μg/kg/min), or etomidate.

9. Deep hypothermia to 18°C permits 1 hour of circulatory arrest.
10. Intra-op angiography—useful when available to determine if clip placement is adequate.
11. Asymptomatic aneurysms > 10 mm should probably be treated unless there are serious medical issues (advanced age, etc.).

J. Specific aneurysms

1. Cavernous ICA aneurysm
   a. Usually does not require surgical intervention because hemorrhage is not intradural and the tendency to rupture is low
   b. Signs/Symptoms—may be caused by mass effect or carotid–cavernous fistula (CCF) formation after rupture
   c. Exposure via pterional approach with proximal control by cervical carotid exposure (or endovascular approach)
2. Carotid cave segment ICA aneurysm
   a. Exposure via pterional approach with proximal control by cervical carotid exposure
   b. Drilling of the anterior clinoid is usually necessary.
   c. Mostly extradural but may have an intradural component and should be treated on the basis of size and history of rupture
3. Ophthalmic artery aneurysm
   a. Exposure via pterional approach with proximal control by cervical carotid exposure (perform first)
   b. Aneurysm usually lies directly under the optic nerve and points up from the ICA.
   c. Usually safe to clip the parent vessel (ophthalmic artery) if necessary
   d. Anterior clinoid process may need to be drilled to the optic strut, the optic strut removed, and the falciform ligament cut
   e. If bilateral, both can be approached from one side.
   f. Superior hypophyseal artery aneurysms are just distal to the ophthalmic artery, are approached the same way, and usually point down.

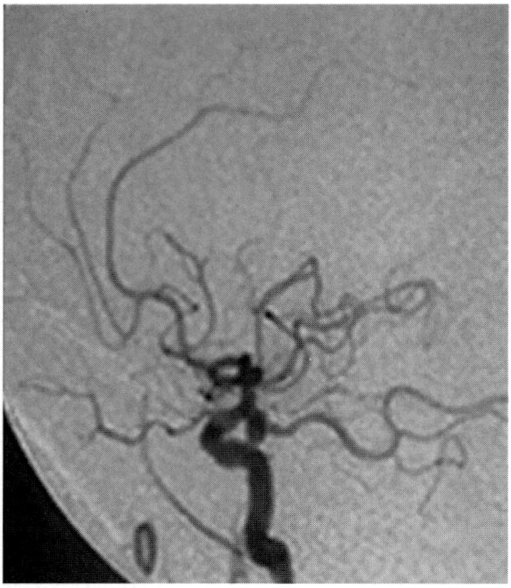

Figure 10–7 Posterior communicating artery aneurysm; lateral angiogram. (With permission from Citow JS. Neuropathology and Neuroradiology: A Review. *New York, NY: Thieme Medical Publishers; 2001:164, Fig. 209B.)*

4. Posterior communicating (PCOM) artery aneurysm
   a. Signs/Symptoms—presentation may be with a dilated pupil with spared ocular movements (Figs. 10–7, 10–8, 10–9).
   b. Exposure via pterional approach
   c. Aneurysm usually points laterally.
   d. Sundt encircling clip should be available in case of tearing of the aneurysm from the ICA.

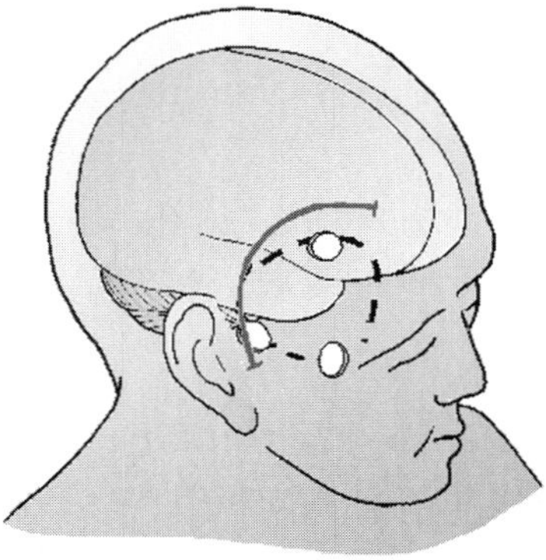

Figure 10–8 Pterional craniotomy incision.

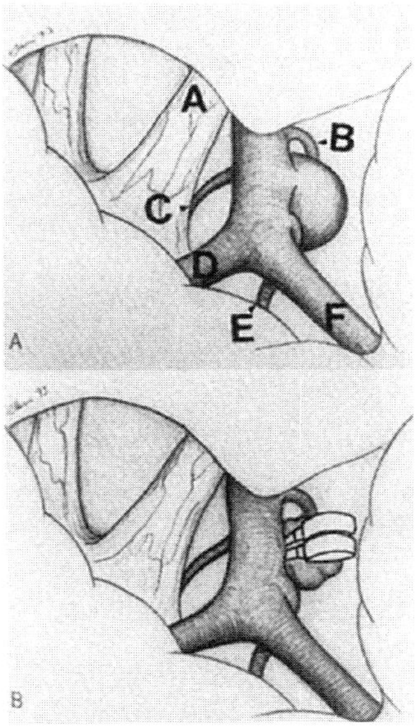

Figure 10–9 Posterior communicating (PCOM) artery aneurysm exposure: (A) optic nerve, (B) PCOM, (C) superior hypophyseal artery, (D) anterior cerebral artery, (E) anterior choroidal artery, (F) middle cerebral artery. (Alleyne, p.19 question 109–114 diagrams with a table.) (With permission from Citow JS. Comprehensive Neurosurgical Board Review. *New York, NY: Thieme Medical Publishers; 2000:436, Fig. 5–1.)*

e. Avoid retracting the temporal lobe until near the end of the exposure because this may precipitate hemorrhage.

5. Anterior choroidal artery aneurysm—exposure via pterional approach
6. ICA bifurcation aneurysm—exposure via pterional approach
7. Middle cerebral artery aneurysm—exposure via pterional approach working from proximal to distal or by splitting the sylvian fissure and working distal to proximal
8. Anterior communicating artery aneurysm—exposure via pterional approach with possible resection of the gyrus rectus.
9. Distal anterior cerebral artery aneurysm—exposure via pterional approach if proximal at the orbitofrontal artery but usually it requires an interhemispheric approach
10. Posterior cerebral artery (PCA) aneurysm
    a. Exposure via subtemporal approach
    b. Subtemporal craniotomy—performed by making a horseshoe incision around the superior pinna
    c. Temporal lobe is retracted superiorly to expose the tentorial edge.

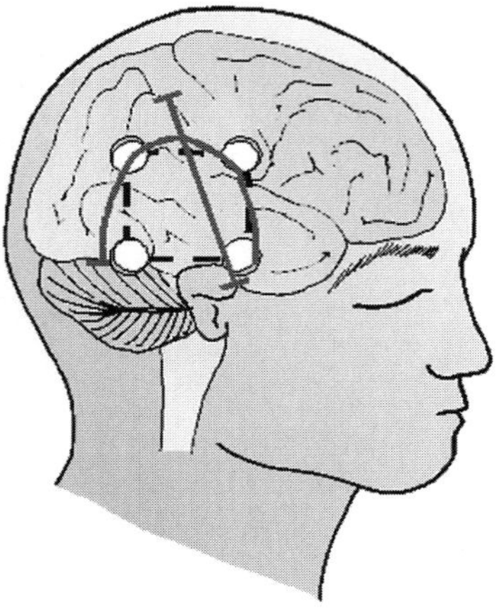

Figure 10–10 Subtemporal craniotomy incision.

d. Tentorium should be divided anterior to the trochlear nerve for basilar artery aneurysms and posterior for PCA aneurysms.

e. PCA is identified and followed to the aneurysm (Fig. 10–10).

11. Basilar artery apex aneurysm

a. Exposure is via pterional approach (used by Yasergil), subtemporal approach (used by Drake), or half-and-half approach (used by Heros).

b. Frontotemporal-orbito-zygomatic exposure can be added to the pterional approach to improve the exposure.

c. Pterional approach usually uses avenue between ICA and cranial nerve III either anterior or posterior to PCOM

d. Path between optic nerve and ICA is seldom used, although it might be considered for higher aneurysms.

e. Aneurysm > 5 mm below the posterior clinoid—consider a path between cranial nerve III and IV or V and VI.

f. Subtemporal approach may be preferred if aneurysm is more than a few millimeters below posterior clinoid process and pointing posteriorly.

g. Liliequist's membrane is between interpeduncular and chiasmatic cisterns.

h. Endovascular coiling is a reasonable option, though the recurrence rate is 20%.

i. Giant basilar arteries may be treated with clipping during circulatory arrest, Hunterian ligation, or endovascular coiling (though the mass effect is not reduced).

12. Midbasilar artery (AICA) aneurysms

a. Exposure via transpetrosal approach in lateral position with presigmoid supra- and infratentorial exposure with division of superior petrosal sinus.

b. Anterior petrosectomy exposes 5–15 mm below the posterior clinoid process.

c. Approach on the side contralateral to the aneurysm.

13. Vertebrobasilar junction aneurysms

a. Exposure via a presigmoid approach with posterior petrosectomy.

b. This approach exposes lesions > 17 mm below the posterior clinoid process (middle and lower clivus).

14. Posterior inferior cerebellar artery (PICA) aneurysms—exposure is via a suboccipital retrosigmoid craniotomy possibly with a C1 hemilaminectomy.

15. Giant aneurysms (> 2.5 cm)

a. Signs/Symptoms—by mass effect or emboli

b. Treatment—surgical clipping, trapping, or Hunterian proximal ligation possibly with bypass

c. Prior to placing a Selverstone clamp, test collateral flow with baloon occlusion and Alcock's test.

16. Traumatic aneurysms

a. Cause—usually due to penetrating trauma involving the interhemispheric or sylvian fissure

b. Treatment—open trapping or balloon occlusion at the skull base

17. Mycotic aneurysms

a. Cause—most often due to streptococcus associated with bacterial endocarditis.

b. Treatment—6 weeks of antibiotics

i. If aneurysm still present, surgical clipping/trapping is needed.

ii. Follow patient with angiograms at 1, 3, 6, and 12 months.

iii. Avoid anticoagulation

K. Complications

1. Vasospasm

a. Occurs from days 4 to 14 (peak at day 7) as blood breakdown products irritate vessels near subarachnoid hemorrhage

b. Risk is assessed by Fisher grade

c. Evaluation—transcranial Doppler (> 200 indicates spasm), cerebral blood flow studies, and angiography.

d. Prevention—nimodipine 60 mg SL q4h.

i. Some studies suggest using intraventricular t-PA 1 mg/d until the blood is dissolved.

e. Treatment—triple-H therapy: hypervolemia (CVP 12 and wedge 20), hypertension, and hemodilution (if HCT < 30%, O_2 delivery impaired)

i. Maintain blood pressure at lowest level where the deficit disappears.

ii. Refractory cases may be treated with intra-arterial papaverine or angioplasty.

2. Hydrocephalus

a. Many surgeons insert a ventricular catheter at the time of surgical clipping to minimize brain retraction and to monitor intracranial pressure after surgery to determine if a shunt will be needed.

b. If catheter must be inserted before surgery for massive hydrocephalus, it should be set to drain at 15 cm of water to prevent detamponading of the aneurysm.

c. 30% of patients with aneurysmal subarachnoid hemorrhage will require a shunt.

3. Hyponatremia—usually due to cerebral salt wasting (CSW) by atrial naturetic factor (patients are hypovolemic) vs SIADH (normo- or hypervolemic)

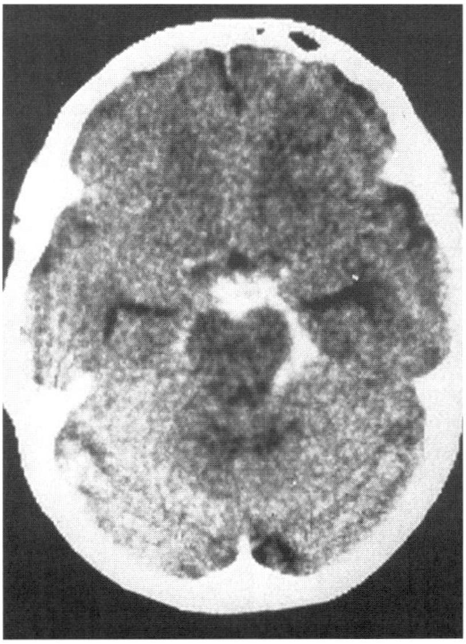

Figure 10–11 Benign perimesencephalic hemorrhage. Computed tomography demonstrates typical subarachnoid hemorrhage extending into the left ambient cistern (angiogram was normal). (With permission from Citow JS. Neuropathology and Neuroradiology: A Review. *New York, NY: Thieme Medical Publishers; 2001:171, Fig. 225.)*

a. Treatment for CSW—fluid replacement with normal saline

b. Treatment for SIADH—fluid restriction

4. Post-op focal deficit—evaluate with angiography (to check for parent vessel occlusion) and CT (to search for clot) and then possibly surgery for clip adjustment.

L. Benign perimesencephalic hemorrhage—subarachnoid hemorrhage in prepontine or perimesencephalic cisterns possibly due to rupture of a small vein.

a. Evaluation—CT, angiogram, MRA

i. Consider repeat angiogram in 10 days if blood not at the perimesencephalic cistern or anterior brain stem.

ii. Also consider cervical spine MRI to rule out AVM.

b. Seldom recurs (Fig. 10–11)

IV. Vascular Malformations

A. Arteriovenous malformation hemorrhage

1. Mortality—1%/y and 10%/bleed

2. Morbidity—2.5%/y and 40%/bleed

3. Initial hemorrhage rate—4%/y

4. Rehemorrhage rate—6%/y × 6 months then 3%/y

B. Spetzler–Martin grading scale

Size—< 3 cm (1), 3–6 cm (2), > 6 cm (3).

Eloquent location—noneloquent (0), eloquent (1).

Venous drainage—superficial (0), deep (1).

Total—1 and 2 (95% good outcome), 3 (84%), 4 (73%), 5 (69%).

C. Treatment

1. Surgery

a. Identify and ligate feeding arteries with care taken to avoid sacrificing vessels just passing through.

b. Avoid entering the malformation during dissection and ligate the draining veins as the last step.

c. Perform surgery 1 week after embolization.

d. To decrease the likelihood of normal perfusion pressure breakthrough, which can cause post-op edema and hemorrhage, try 3 days of pre-op treatment with propanolol 20 mg PO q.i.d.

e. Surgical risks

i. Consider Spetzler-Martin grading scale

ii. Aneurysms (feeding, draining, or intranidal)

iii. High- or low-flow AVMs

iv. Recent hemorrhage—may make the dissection plane more obvious

v. 10% of AVMs have aneurysms.

vi. Higher risk of hemorrhage with intranidal aneurysms and venous stenosis (Fig. 10–12)

2. Radiation

a. Stereotactic radiosurgery—proven useful for lesions < 3 cm

b. Complete obliteration rate—80% (only 50% for larger lesions)

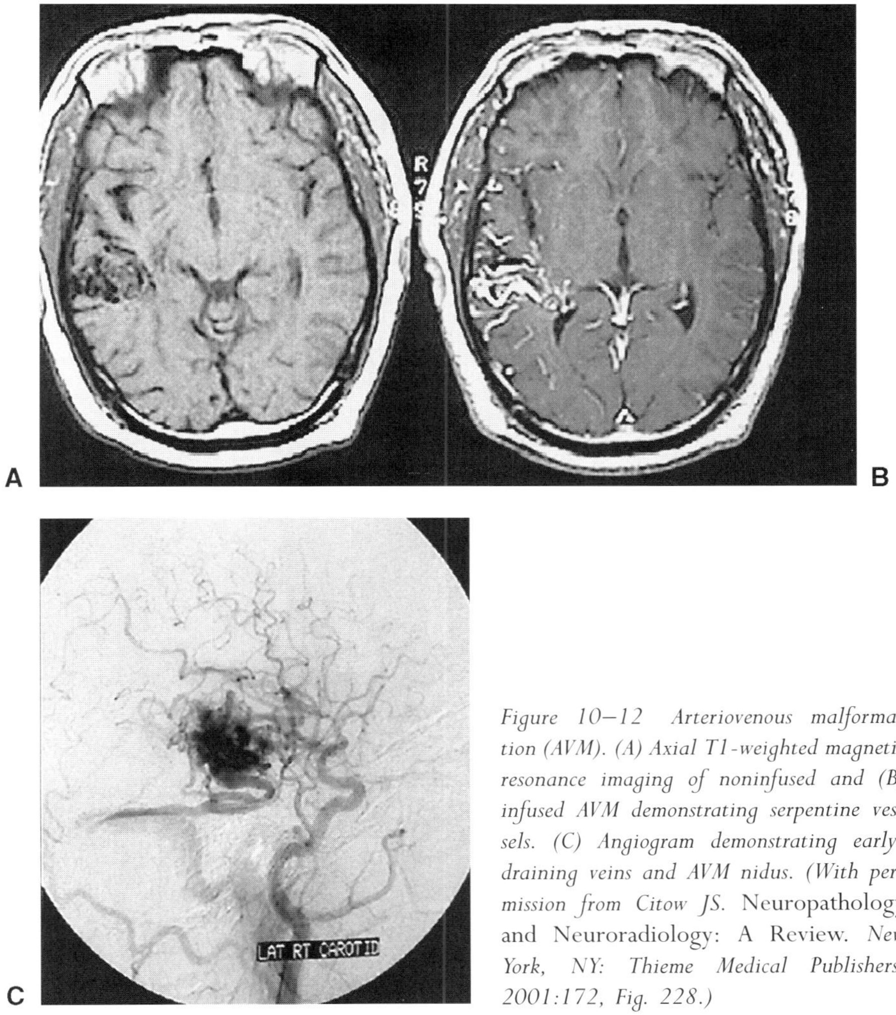

Figure 10–12 Arteriovenous malformation (AVM). (A) Axial T1-weighted magnetic resonance imaging of noninfused and (B) infused AVM demonstrating serpentine vessels. (C) Angiogram demonstrating early-draining veins and AVM nidus. (With permission from Citow JS. Neuropathology and Neuroradiology: A Review. *New York, NY: Thieme Medical Publishers; 2001:172, Fig. 228.)*

c. 18-month delay before vessels become occluded and hemorrhage risk decreases

d. Risk of increased neurological deficit from therapy is 3%

e. Incomplete obliteration—radiosurgery can be repeated.

f. Consider for deep lesions or around eloquent cortex

g. Radiosurgery best performed 30 days after embolization

3. Endovascular embolization
    a. Only useful as an adjuvant to other therapies
    b. Risk of complications (i.e., CVA)—5%
    c. Most useful for dural AVF, cavernous carotid fistula, or vein of Galen malformation

D. Angiographically occult AVM (cryptic)—due to either a small feeding vessel (beyond the resolution of angiography) or a vessel compressed by a hemorrhage

E. Cavernous malformation
1. Not visualized on angiogram
2. Frequently associated with seizures
3. 50% are multiple.
4. Hemorrhage—risk is as low as 0.07%/y.
5. Treatment
    a. Surgery if symptomatic
    b. Radiosurgery not shown to be of benefit
    c. Brain stem cavernous malformations have higher risk of hemorrhage and should be resected if there have been two or more hemorrhages (though some surgeons suggest resection after only one).
    d. Be sure to open brain stem where malformation is closest to the surface.
    e. An approach superior and lateral to the facial colliculus has been used.

F. Dural AVM—actually an AVF (arteriovenous fistula) because there is no nidus
1. May arise from carotid or vertebral circulation (esp. occipital artery) and drain into dural sinuses (usually the transverse–sigmoid junction).
2. Believed to be acquired by collateral revascularization after sinus thrombosis.
3. Signs/Symptoms—pulsatile tinnitus, bruits, headaches
4. Hemorrhage—risk is 4%/y

5. Most behave benignly, but hemorrhage risk increases with cortical drainage or lesions in tentorial apex (as high as 80%) or anterior fossa (70%).
6. Treatment
   a. Initially—endovascular embolization of the fistulous connection
   b. Blockage of arterial feeders has relatively low success rate because there is frequently vessel recruitment
      i. If this fails, consider surgery to skeletonize the sinus (Fig. 10–13A,B).

G. Cavernous-carotid fistula

1. May either be posttraumatic or spontaneous
2. Connection may be from ICA to cavernous sinus (high flow) or meningeal branches of ICA or ECA to cavernous sinus (low flow)
3. Signs/Symptoms—chemosis, proptosis, bruit, eye pain, visual loss, ophthalmoplegia.
4. 50% of low-flow lesions spontaneously thrombose.

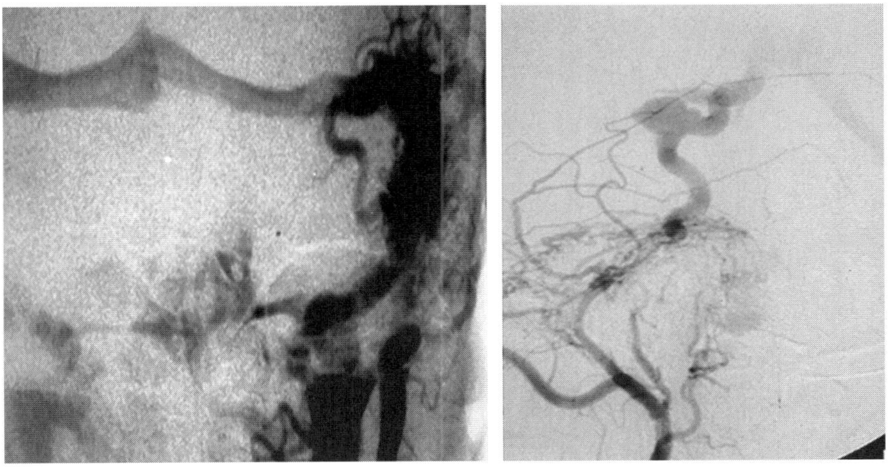

Figure 10–13 Dural arteriovenous malformation (AVM). (A)Anteroposterior and (B) lateral external carotid artery (ECA) angiograms demonstrate supply from the ECA with early filling into the sigmoid sinus. (With permission from Citow JS. Neuropathology and Neuroradiology: A Review. *New York, NY: Thieme Medical Publishers; 2001:175, Fig. 232.)*

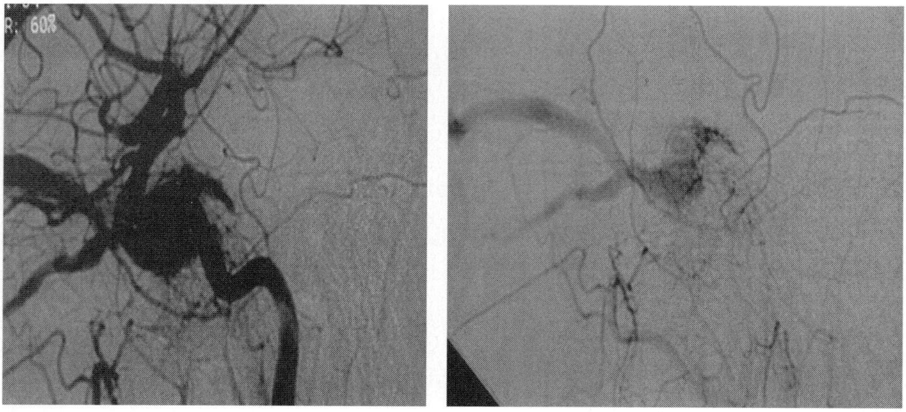

Figure 10–14 Cavernous-carotid fistula. (A) Lateral angiograms of the common carotid artery demonstrating early filling of the cavernous sinus with dilated superior and inferior ophthalmic veins and (B) of the external carotid artery (ECA) demonstrating filling from the ECA. (With permission from Citow JS. Comprehensive Neurosurgical Board Review. *New York, NY: Thieme; 2000:441, Fig. 5–2.)*

5. Low-flow lesions may be observed if vision is normal and intraocular pressure < 25 (though frequent visual exams are needed).
6. Treatment
    a. Initially—balloon occlusion
        i. Through ICA to fistula
        ii. Two balloons to trap the ICA
        iii. Or cavernous sinus occlusion via superior ophthalmic vein.
    b. Before trapping the ICA, test tolerance with a balloon occlusion under controlled hypotension to SBP 80 mm Hg and evaluate for symptoms or evaluate with SPECT scan to determine ischemia.
    c. If patient cannot tolerate trapping, perform ECA–ICA bypass (Fig. 10–14A,B)

V. Neonatal Hemorrhage

A. Germinal matrix hemorrhage

1. Located in subependymal region and may extend into ventricle
2. Due to impaired autoregulation before 34 weeks and found in 40% of children born before 35 weeks

3. Frequency increases with asphyxia due to hypertension and hypercapnea.
4. Prevention may be accomplished with indomethacin to close patent ductus arteriosus and increase pO_2.
5. 75% of grade II hemorrhages have normal IQ
6. Full-term children usually develop intraventricular hemorrhages.

B. Evaluation—ultrasound, OFC (35% develop hydrocephalus), CSF (protein < 100 may resolve spontaneously)

C. Treatment
1. Acetazolamide
2. Daily removal of CSF with ventricular taps (< 800 g)
3. Serial LPs (> 800 g)
4. Ventricular access device (> 1100 g)
5. Amount of CSF to remove is 10mL/kg/tap or until the manometer lowers to 3 cm water (tap before it exceeds 10 cm water)
6. Consider VP shunt if > 2500 g (earlier may cause necrotizing enterocolitis)

CHAPTER 11

Head Trauma

I. Glasgow Coma Scale (GCS)

A. Eye opening—none (1), to pain (2), to voice (3), spontaneously (4)

B. Verbal output—none (1), sounds (2), words (3), disoriented (4), oriented (5)

C. Motor function—none (1), extensor posturing (2), flexor posturing (3), withdrawal from pain (4), localizing (5), following commands (6)

II. Head Trauma Grading—severe (GCS 3–8), moderate (GCS 9–12), mild (GCS 13–15)

III. Good Outcomes—GCS 3–6 (8%), 7–8 (41%), 9–12 (81%)

A. Outcome worse if SBP < 90 mm Hg or $pO_2 < 60$ mm Hg

IV. Intracranial Pressure Monitor—place if GCS < 8 with an abnormal CT

V. Cerebral Perfusion Pressure—maintain > 70; try to keep ICP < 20 mm Hg

VI. ICP Control

A. CSF drainage

B. Mannitol—1 g/kg bolus and 0.25 g/kg q6h.

1. Check serum osmolarity q6h and hold mannitol if < 320 to avoid acute tubular necrosis.
2. Maintain euvolemia and normokalemia.
3. Avoid mannitol with CHF or renal failure.

C. Sedation and paralytics

D. Pentobarbital coma

1. Lowers ICP and $CMRO_2$
2. Decreases free radicals
3. Produces hypotension by decreasing sympathetic tone and causing myocardial depression
4. Increase dose until burst suppression achieved on EEG.
5. Insert Swan-Ganz catheter and NG tube (for hyperalimentation)
6. Dose—thiopental 5 mg/kg IV over 10 minutes, 5 mg/kg/h × 24 hours, and 2.5 mg/kg/h to control ICP/EEG (level 6–8.5 mg/dL)
7. Consider propofol 10 μg/kg/min up to 170 μg/kg/min in place of barbiturates.

VII. Other Measures

A. Fever control—cooling blanket and rectal Tylenol

B. Carafate or Pepcid

C. DVT prophylaxis—TED hose, SCD, and heparin SQ

D. Tube feeds after 3 days

VIII. Skull Fracture—elevate if open (also needs antibiotics), or if there is a CSF leak, an underlying clot, or a fragment depressed more than the thickness of the skull

IX. Sinus Wall Fracture—treat with 10 days of ciprofloxacin and surgical repair.

X. Epidural Hematoma

A. May watch if < 1 cm (be very careful)

B. Use question mark or linear incision but be sure to expose low enough to reach foramen spinosum (middle meningeal artery).

C. Consider placement of ICP monitor if there is also cerebral edema.

D. Have blood available.

XI. Gunshot Wound

A. Monitor ABCs and address other injuries.

B. Shave around the wound, irrigate and debride, and finally staple the wound closed.

C. Use Dilantin (or fosphenytoin), Ancef, and tetanus toxoid.

D. Consider an angiogram to rule out vessel injury for lesions crossing the sylvian fissure or interhemispheric fissure.

E. Don't operate if GCS 3–4 or 5–6 without a mass lesion.

XII. Facial Palsy—if partial or worsening, consider ENT decompression; surgery rarely needed

XIII. Tension Pneumocephalus—when nitrous oxide not stopped before dural closure

XIV. Posttraumatic Leptomeningeal Cyst (Growing Skull Fracture)—fix with craniotomy around lesion and dural repair.

XV. Benign Subdural Collections of Infancy—most resolve spontaneously.

XVI. Cephalohematoma

A. Subgaleal hematoma—does not calcify, resolves spontaneously.

B. Subperiosteal hematoma

1. Occurs mainly in newborns and is limited by sutures
2. 80% resorb spontaneously.
3. May calcify
4. Surgical evacuation for cosmetics is performed after 6 weeks.

XVII. Child Abuse—search for retinal hemorrhages, long bone fractures, subdural hematomas (especially interhemispheric), and non-parietal skull fractures.

XVIII. Concussion—transient altered mentation or loss of consciousness following head trauma.

A. For management guideline for sports-related concussions see Tables 11–1, 11–2, 11–3, 11–4.

Table 11.1 Concussion grading

Grade	**Cantu system***	**★AAN system***
1 (mild)	A. PTA < 30 mins B. no LOC	A. transient confusion B. no LOC C. symptoms resolve in < 15 mins
2 (moderate)	A. LOC < 5 mins, or B. PTA > 30 mins	as above, but symptoms last > 15 mins (still no LOC) (PTA is common)
3 (severe)	A. LOC ≥ 5 mins, or B. PTA ≥ 24 hrs	any LOC, whether brief (seconds) or prolonged

* abbreviations: LOC = loss of consciousness; PTA = posttraumatic amnesia

Table 11.2 Cerebral contraindications for return to contact sports

A. persistent postconcussion symptoms
B. permanent CNS sequelae from head injury (e.g. organic dementia, hemiplegia, homonymous hemianopsia)
C. hydrocephalus
D. spontaneous SAH from any cause
E. symptomatic (neurologic or pain producing) abnormalities about the foramen magnum (e.g. Chiari malformation)

TABLE 11.3 RECOMMENDATIONS FOR MULTIPLE SPORTS-RELATED CONCUSSIONS IN THE SAME SEASON

Concusion No.	Severity	Guidelines to be met before return to competition
2	mild	1 week*
	moderate or severe	1 month* + normal CT or MRI†
3	mild	most consider this a season ending injury and recommend CT or MRI†
	moderate	season ending injury, consideration for ending all participation in contact sports
2	severe	season ending injury, consideration for ending all participation in contact sports

* without symptoms at rest and with exertion (*see text*)

† if any acute abnormalities on CT/MRI: terminate season. Consider ending all participation in contact sports

TABLE 11.4 MANAGEMENT OPTIONS FOLLOWING CONCUSSION

AAN grade	Management options[8]
1 (mild)	A. remove from contest
	B. examine q 5 mins for amnesia or postconcussive symptoms*
	C. may return to contest if symptoms clear within 15 mins
2 (moderate)	A. remove from contest
	B. disallow return that day
	C. examine on-site frequently for signs of evolving intracranial pathology
	D. reexamination the next day by a trained individual
	E. CT or MRI if H/A or other symptoms worsen or last > 1 week†
	F. return to practice after 1 full week without symptoms*
3 (severe)	A. ambulance transport from field to E/R if still unconscious or for concerning signs (C-spine precautions if indicated)
	B. emergent neuro exam. Neuroimaging as appropriate
	C. may go home with head-injury instructions if normal findings at time of initial neuro exam
	D. admit to hospital for any signs of pathology or for continued abnormal mental status

Continues

TABLE 11.4 *Continued*

AAN grade	Management options[8]
	E. assess neuro status daily until all symptoms have stabilized or resolved F. prolonged unconsciousness, persistent mental status alterations, worsening post-concussion symptoms, or abnormalities on neurologic exam → urgent neurosurgical evaluation or transfer to a trauma center G. after brief (< 1 minute) grade 3 concussion, do not return to practice until asymptomatic for 1 full week* H. after prolonged (> 1 minute) grade 3 concussion, return to practice only after 2 full weeks without symptoms*‡ I. CT or MRI if H/A or other symptoms worsen or last > 1 week†

* evaluation at rest and with exertion (*see text*)

† season is terminated for that player if CT/MRI shows edema, contusion, or other acute intracranial pathology. Return to play in any contact sports in the future should be seriously discouraged

‡ some experts also require a normal CT scan

CHAPTER 12

Spine Trauma

I. Spinal Shock

A. Loss of sympathetic tone and muscle paralysis cause venous pooling with hypotension (usually occur with injuries above T7).

B. Loss of voluntary and reflex movements as well as sensation after a spinal cord injury; may last as long as 2 weeks; priapism is a bad sign.

II. Hypotension

A. Causes—hypovolemia, myocardial dysfunction, or loss of sympathetic tone

B. Treatment

1. Loss of sympathetic tone—Levophed (norepinephrine), phenylephrine (may cause reflex bradycardia), or dopamine to maintain SBP > 90 mm Hg
2. Prevent pulmonary edema from overhydration.
3. Use atropine for bradycardia.

III. Initial Management

A. Immobilize with cervical collar and backboard.

B. Address ABCs (airway, breathing, circulation); consider nasotracheal intubation if no suspected cribriform plate trauma.

C. Insert NG tube (ileus common), Foley catheter, and A-line.

D. Initiate DVT prophylaxis with TED hose, sequential compression devices (SCDs), and SQ heparin or Lovenox.

E. Watch for hypothermia and electrolyte abnormalities.

IV. Radiological Evaluation

A. Cervical, thoracic, and lumbar spine x-rays; CXR; KUB; and pelvic x-ray

B. No need to perform flexion–extension x-ray if > 3.5 mm subluxation because there is almost certainly instability

C. Children < 4 years may have pseudospread of the atlas on AP 2–8 mm (a fracture must be determined by CT).

D. Children may also have 3 mm of subluxation at C2–3 up to 10 years.

V. Solumedrol (Methylprednisolone) Protocol

A. Traumatic spinal cord dysfunction—medication must be started within 8 hours of injury.

B. Dose—30 mg/kg over 45 minutes, wait 15 minutes, then 5.4 mg/kg/h over 23 hours

C. Third NASCAS study suggests that if steroids are started within 3 hours of injury, they should be continued for 24 hours; if started from 3–8 hours after injury, they should be continued for 48 hours.

VI. Traction

A. Avoid in cases of atlanto-occipital dislocation, type 2 or 3 hangman's fractures, or children < 3 years

B. Consider MRI before initiating traction to make sure there is not a herniated disk that may be pulled into the spinal cord (rare occurrence).

C. Place Gardner-Wells tongs with pins 2.5 fingerbreadths above the pinna; for neutral position above the EAM, for flexion 2 cm posterior, and for extension 2 cm anterior.

   1. Tighten pins daily for 3 days to 60 lbs (pin indicator 1 cm beyond surface).

2. Avoid using traction weight > 40–50 lbs.
3. Obtain frequent x-rays to evaluate alignment and make sure that the disk spaces do not exceed 10 mm and the occipital condyle–C1 lateral mass spaces do not exceed 5 mm.
4. Halo pins should be placed while the eyes are closed to 8 lbs/inch and the bars tightened to 30 lbs/inch.
5. Dislocation reduction is best performed with fluoroscopy to save time.
6. Avoid raising the head preventing the patient from seeing the ground, but avoid overflexion preventing the patient from swallowing.
7. Use pin care with half-strength hydrogen peroxide and bacitracin ointment t.i.d.
8. Complications—epidural hematoma, skull fracture, herniated disk, occipito-atlantal dislocation, infection

VII. Spinal Cord Levels—to determine the location of a spinal cord level in relation to the vertebral level, subtract 2 from T2–10 to be at the spinal cord level.

A. Bones of T11–L1 are over the spinal cord levels L1–5, S1–5, and C1 (Fig. 12–1).

VIII. Complete Injury

A. No voluntary movement, sensation, or sphincter control below injured spinal cord level

B. Priapism may occur from lack of sympathetic input.

C. Watch for hypotension and bradycardia.

D. Autonomic dysreflexia may occur with an injury above T6; includes an exaggerated sympathetic response with hypertension, sweating, and flushing.

1. May be stimulated by bowel or bladder emptying.
2. Treatment—HOB elevation, Nipride or phentolamine, Valium, and maintaining an empty bladder and bowel

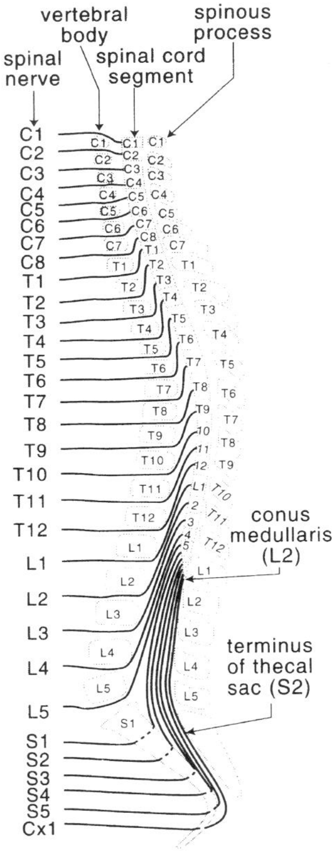

Figure 12–1 Spinal cord levels. (With permission from Greenberg MS. Handbook of Neurosurgery. *5th ed. New York, NY: Thieme Medical Publishers; 2001:695, Fig. 25–1.)*

IX. Incomplete Injuries

A. Central cord syndrome—the most frequent incomplete injury

1. Cause—hyperextension, usually with preexisting cervical stenosis
2. Signs/Symptoms—weakness (more in the UE than LE because the UE fibers are medial in the corticospinal and spinothalamic tracts), and various sensory and sphincter dysfunction.
3. Treatment
   a. No evidence that early surgery improves outcome
   b. Decompression performed 1–3 weeks after injury to prevent recurrence and instability

B. Anterior cord syndrome

1. Cause—anterior spinal artery CVA causing decreased motor function and loss of pain and temperature sensation, with sparing of proprioception
    a. Frequently associated with aortic dissection
2. Prognosis—poor

C. Brown-Séquard's syndrome—hemicord injury with ipsilateral motor and light touch/proprioception deficit with contralateral pain/temperature deficit
1. Cause—usually a penetrating injury
2. Prognosis if the deficit is partial—relatively good

D. Posterior cord injury—causes only paresthesias and rarely occurs

X. SCIWORA

A. Cause—usually occurs in children due to ligamentous flexibility

B. Evaluation—inpatient with MRI and flexion–extension x-rays

C. Treatment—collar should be worn for 3 weeks and sports avoided for 3 months

XI. Cervical Fracture Stability

A. Classical classification scheme—by White and Punjabi.

B. Nondisplaced fracture—assess stability with flexion–extension x-rays.
1. Unstable—place in collar (or other orthosis) for 6–12 weeks and assess fusion at that point with another flexion–extension x-ray (various injury types are discussed later)
2. No instability on the dynamic x-ray—no collar needed; however, study may be insufficient because cervical muscle spasm may prevent adequate motion to demonstrate instability
    a. Study questionable—keep patient in collar and repeat study in 2 weeks
3. Ligamentous instability—present if > 3.5 mm of subluxation or > 11 degrees of angulation.

a. These injuries usually require surgical stabilization because only 10–15% heal with immobilization.

XII. Atlanto-Occipital Dislocation

A. Joint stabilized mainly by tectorial membrane (posterior longitudinal ligament from C2 to occiput) and alar ligaments (from dens to C1 and occiput)

B. Distance from occipital condyle to superior facet of atlas should be < 5 mm.

C. Distance from basion to tip of dens should be < 5 mm in adults and < 10 mm in children.

D. Power's ratio—(anterior basion to posterior arch of C1):(opisthion to anterior arch) > 1—suggests anterior dislocation (most frequent injury).

E. Type 1 injury is anterior subluxation, type 2 is distraction, type 3 is posterior subluxation (very rare).

F. Treatment

1. Place patient in a halo immediately.
2. Stabilize with occiput–C3 fusion with sublaminar/suboccipital wires and a horseshoe rod ($\frac{3}{8}$ inch Steinmann pin or Omni loop).
3. Lateral mass plates with occipital extension may also be used.
4. If a condylar fracture presses on brain stem, patient should be placed in a halo and treated with transoral decompression followed by posterior fusion.
5. Evaluate for associated vertebral artery dissection with MRA; if present treat with heparin/Coumadin for 3 months (Fig. 12–2).

XIII. Atlantoaxial Dislocation

A. Anterior dislocation

1. Cause—transverse ligament injury or dens fracture
2. Treatment

a. C1–2 fusion using sublaminar wires (i.e., Brook's, Gallie, or Sonntag) or transarticular screws. (See the section on rheumatoid arthritis.)

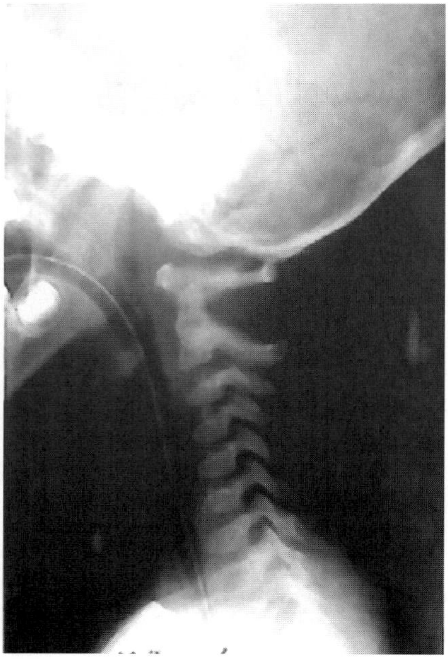

Figure 12–2 Atlanto-occipital and atlantoaxial dislocations. Lateral cervical spine x-ray film demonstrates increased distance from the occiput to the atlas and the atlas to the axis. (With permission from Citow JS. Neuropathology and Neuroradiology: A Review. *New York, NY: Thieme Medical Publishers; 2001:211, Fig. 295.)*

b. Brooks technique—sublaminar wires under both C1 and 2 with two cubes of bone between the laminas.

c. Gallie technique—H-shaped bone graft over C1 and 2 held by a wire sublaminar at C1 and around the spinous process of C2.

d. Dickman and Sonntag technique—similar to Gallie technique with the wire sublaminar under C1 only, but the bone graft is U-shaped and lodged between the laminas of C1 and 2 as well as around the spinous process of C2.

e. Songer titanium cables should be tightened to 30 lbs/inch (Figs. 12–3A–C, 12–4).

B. Rotatory subluxation—occurs in children (often after an upper respiratory infection) or rheumatoid patients.

1. Signs/Symptoms—head tilt, flexion, and rotation

2. Evaluation—CT

3. Treatment—attempt reduction with 7–15 lbs of traction.

a. If reduced—immobilize for 6 weeks and reassess with dynamic studies.

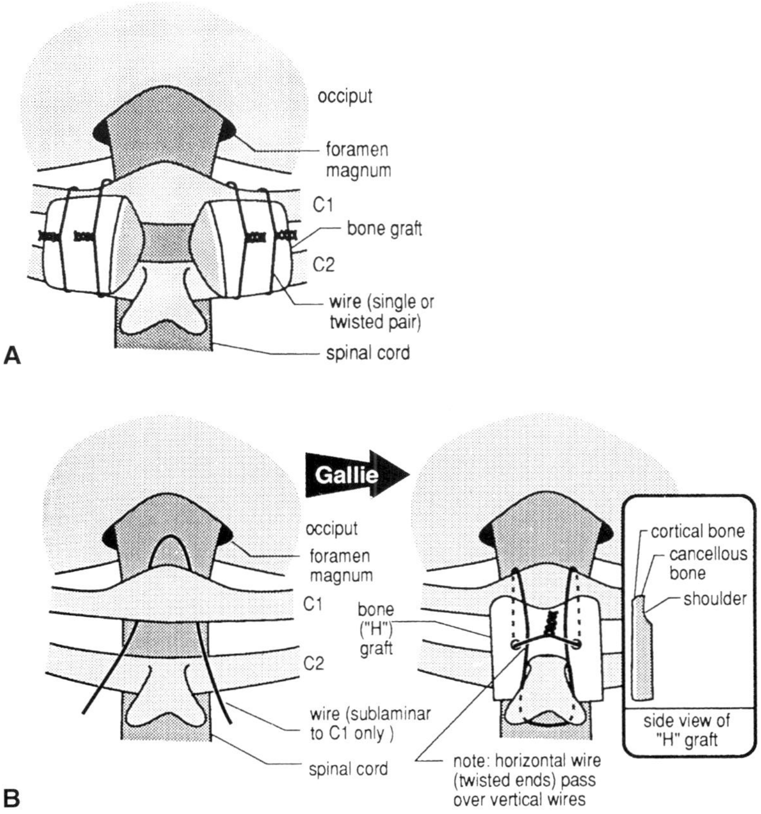

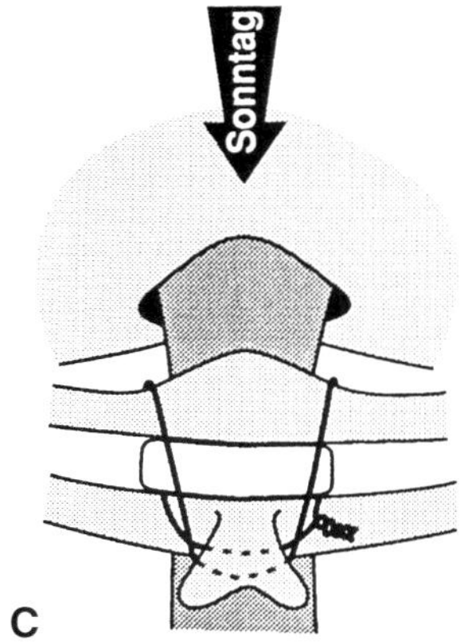

Figure 12–3 *(A) Brooks fusion. (B) Gallie fusion. (C) Sonntag fusion. (With permission from Greenberg MS.* Handbook of Neurosurgery. *3rd ed. Lakeland, FL: Greenberg Graphics, Inc.; 1994:498–499, Figs. 42–2 and 42–3.)*

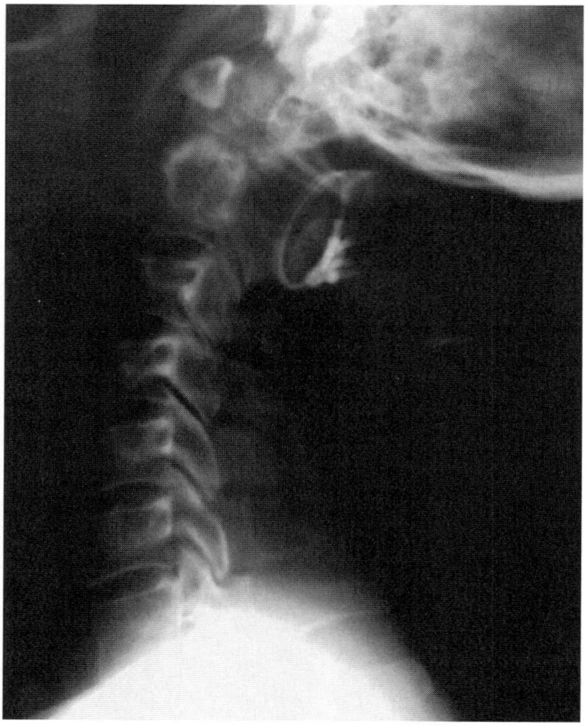

Figure 12–4 Lateral cervical spine x-ray of Brooks fusion.

b. Fuse early at C1–2 if there is anterior subluxation or the transverse atlantal ligament is disrupted (Fig. 12–5A–D).

XIV. C1 Fracture

A. Jefferson's fracture—4-, 3-, or 2-point fractures from axial loading

B. Usually unstable

C. Evaluation—evaluate with open-mouth-view x-ray and CT.

1. According to the rule of Spence, > 7 mm of C1–2 combined overhang on open-mouth x-ray suggests disruption of the transverse atlantal ligament.
2. Ligament can usually be visualized on axial MRI and a disruption determined.

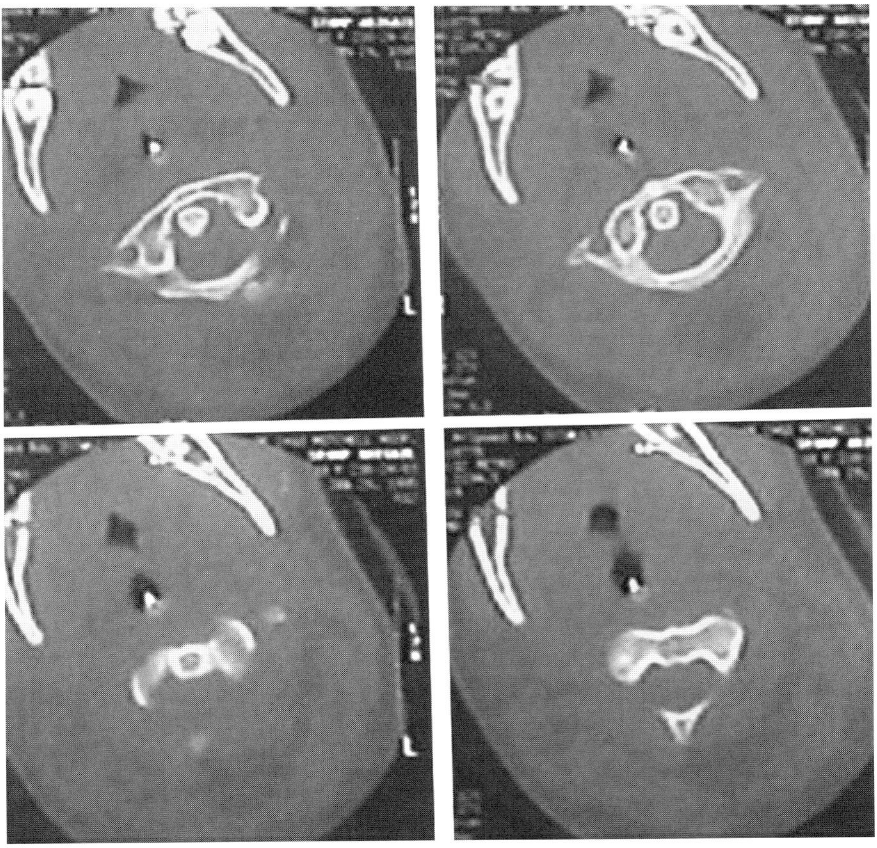

Figure 12–5 Atlantoaxial rotatory subluxation. (A–D) Axial computed tomography demonstrates the 45-degree rotation of the atlas on the axis. (With permission from Citow JS. Neuropathology and Neuroradiology: A Review. *New York, NY: Thieme Medical Publishers; 2001:212, Fig. 297.)*

D. Treatment

1. Fracture of the tubercle connecting the transverse ligament usually heals well with immobilization.
2. If ligament intact—halo or SOMI brace
3. If ligament disrupted—perform occiput–C3 posterior fusion or possibly a C1–2 posterior fusion if arch is stable (Fig. 12–6A–C)

E. C1 and 2 fractures

1. Treatment—according to C2 injury
   a. Hangman's fracture—halo

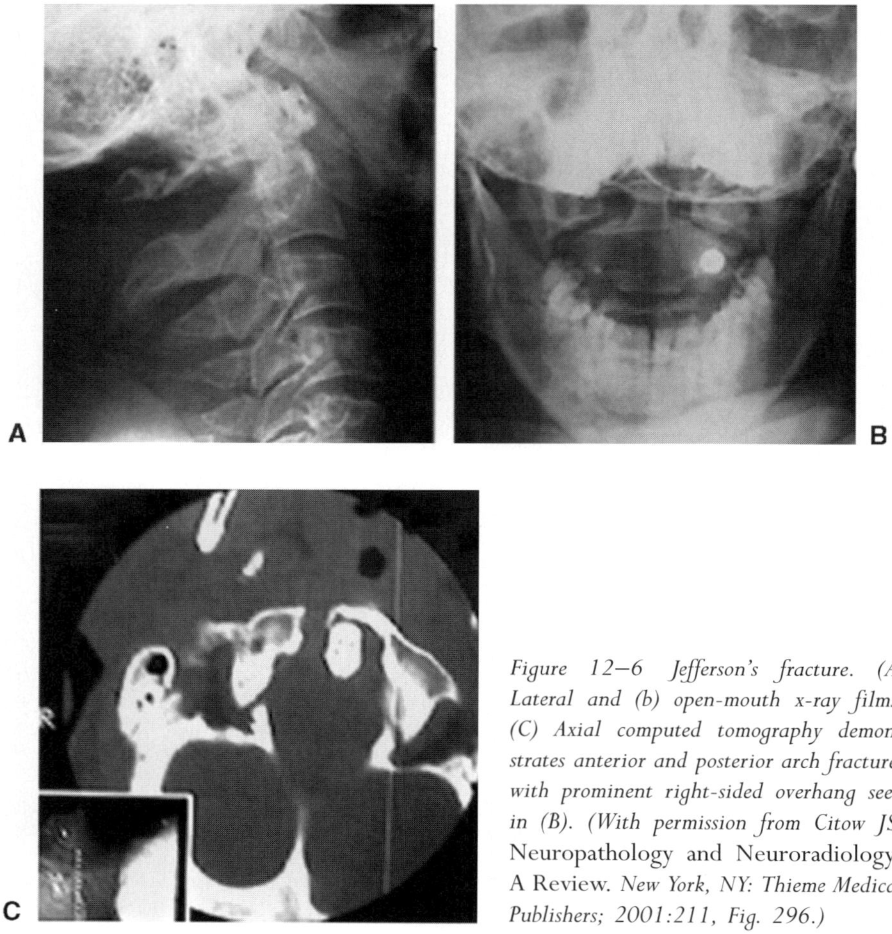

Figure 12–6 Jefferson's fracture. (A) Lateral and (b) open-mouth x-ray films. (C) Axial computed tomography demonstrates anterior and posterior arch fractures with prominent right-sided overhang seen in (B). (With permission from Citow JS. Neuropathology and Neuroradiology: A Review. *New York, NY: Thieme Medical Publishers; 2001:211, Fig. 296.)*

b. Type 2 dens fracture with < 6 mm displacement—halo and > 6 mm displacement (occiput–C2 fusion or C1–2 transarticular screws)

c. Type 3 dens fracture—halo

XV. C2 Fracture

A. Hangman's fracture—pars fracture (spondylolisthesis) between the superior facet process (anterior, in line with the occiput–C1 joint) and inferior facet process (posterior, in line with the other cervical facet joints).

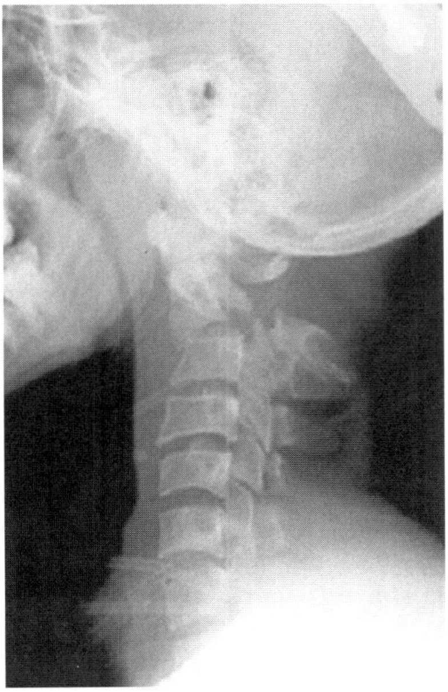

Figure 12–7 Hangman's fracture. Lateral cervical spine x-ray film demonstrates the C2 traumatic spondylolisthesis with anterior angulation. (With permission from Citow JS. Neuropathology and Neuroradiology: A Review. *New York, NY: Thieme Medical Publishers; 2001:213, Fig. 300.)*

1. Cause—Usually from hyperextension and axial loading (not distraction as with judicial hangings of the past)
2. Usually stable and rarely presents with a deficit (Fig. 12–7)
3. Effendi classification (by C2–3 subluxation at the PLL line)

   Type 1—< 3 mm of C2–3 subluxation; treat with SOMI brace 3 months

   Type 2—> 4 mm subluxation or > 11 degrees angulation; reduce with traction then place in a halo or Minerva brace (surgery only if unable to maintain reduction)

   Type 3—C2–3 locked facets with 50% subluxation; treat with an anterior C2–3 fusion or a posterior C1–3 fusion (or C1–2 fusion).

B. Dens fracture—C1–2 joint provides 50% of the motion of the cervical spine.

1. Steele's rule of thirds—at the level of the dens, the spinal canal is filled by thirds of spinal cord, CSF, and dens.
2. Anderson and D'Alonzo classification

a. Type 1—oblique fracture through the tip of the dens (rare), treat with halo

b. Type 2—fracture at base of dens, treat with halo 3 months if < 6 mm displacement or if < 7 years.

   i. Perform fusion if unable to maintain reduction in a halo.

   ii. 30% nonunion rate in a halo, but only 10% if < 6 mm displacement

   iii. Treatment—Surgical options include anterior odontoid screw (maintains range of motion, requires intact transverse ligament, avoid if fracture > 2 weeks old or if patient with barrel chest), posterior transarticular C1–2 screw (need a CT to determine if screws can be placed without vertebral artery injury), or posterior sublaminar wire fusion (Brook's, Gallie, or Sonntag as above) (Fig. 12–8A–C).

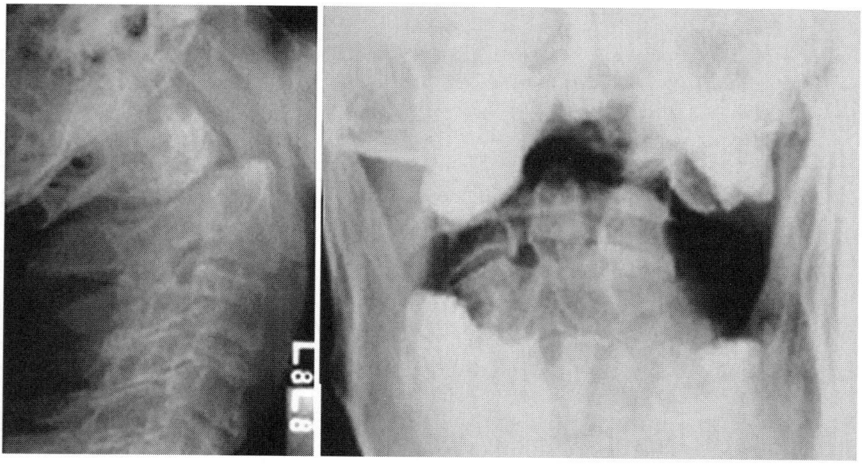

A B

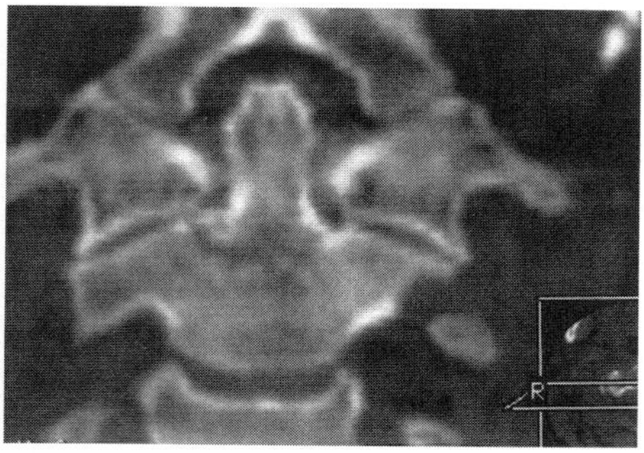

C

Figure 12–8 Odontoid fracture (type 2). (A) Lateral and (B) open-mouth cervical spine x-ray films demonstrate the fracture through the base of the dens with posterior dislocation. (C) Coronal tomography of type 3 dens fracture. (With permission from Citow JS. Neuropathology and Neuroradiology: A Review. *New York, NY: Thieme Medical Publishers; 2001:212, Fig. 298.)*

c. Type 3—fracture through body of axis; stable; treat with a SOMI brace

XVI. Clay Shoveler's Fracture—involves spinous process of C7, C6, or T1.

A. Stable if no associated ligamentous injury

B. No collar needed

XVII. Teardrop Fracture

A. Cause—major flexion injury

B. Produces wedge-shaped fracture on anteroinferior aspect of vertebral body

C. Usually severe ligamentous injury and instability

D. Should be differentiated from a stable compression fracture

E. Treatment—anterior and posterior fusion (with lateral mass plates or interspinous wiring), though a single approach may be sufficient

XVIII. Locked Facets—may be unilateral or bilateral (with > 50% subluxation)

A. Treatment

1. Reduction with traction starting at 3 lbs/level and increasing the weight by 5 lbs every 10 minutes while obtaining x-rays to determine alignment and rule out distraction injury (stop if occipitoatlantal dislocation > 5 mm or disk space > 10 mm)
2. Avoid > 5 lbs per level.
3. Muscle relaxants—may help achieve reduction, but keep patient alert and examinable
4. MRI prior to traction to rule out disk herniation
5. Once patient is reduced, lower the weight to 10 lbs
6. Bilateral facet injury—all patients should be stabilized surgically.
7. Unilateral facet dislocation—many patients will heal in a brace, but surgery should be performed in the presence of radiculopathy or failure to maintain reduction.

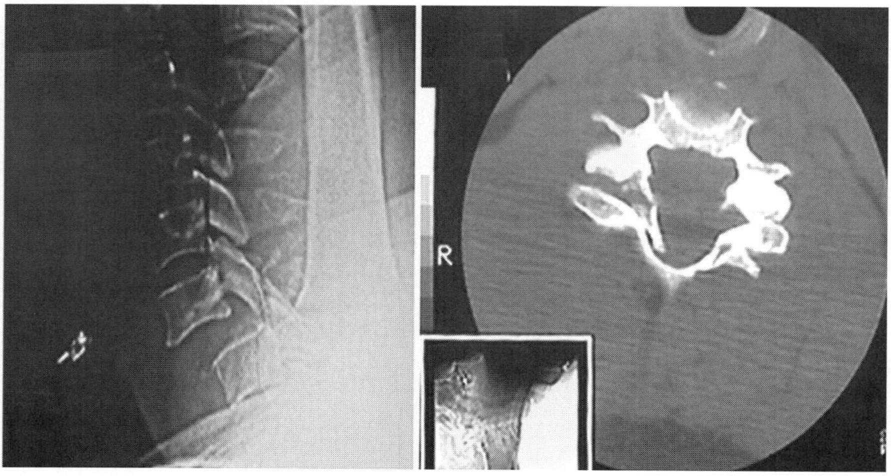

Figure 12–9 Bilateral interfacetal dislocation. (A) Lateral cervical x-ray film and (B) axial computed tomography demonstrates the C6–7 injury with bilateral jumped facets. (With permission from Citow JS. Neuropathology and Neuroradiology: A Review. *New York, NY: Thieme Medical Publishers; 2001:214, Fig. 302.)*

8. Stabilization can be performed anteriorly (with a plate), but the posterior approach (with lateral mass screws and interspinous wires) is preferred.
    a. Lateral mass screws inserted into middle of lateral mass and angled 10–30 degrees laterally and rostrally per x-ray and 14–20 mm deep per x-ray to be bicortical with 3.5 mm screws.
    b. Remember to prepare patient for iliac bone graft
    c. After stabilization, patient is placed in a brace for 6–12 weeks
9. There is often vertebral artery occlusion with facet dislocation (Fig. 12–9A,B).

XIX. Flexion Ligamentous Injury With Posterior Instability—reduce and fuse posteriorly with sublaminar or interspinous wires or lateral mass plates (Fig. 12–10).

XX. Extension Ligamentous Injury or Anterior Compression Fracture—fix anteriorly with cervical diskectomy, fusion, and plating.

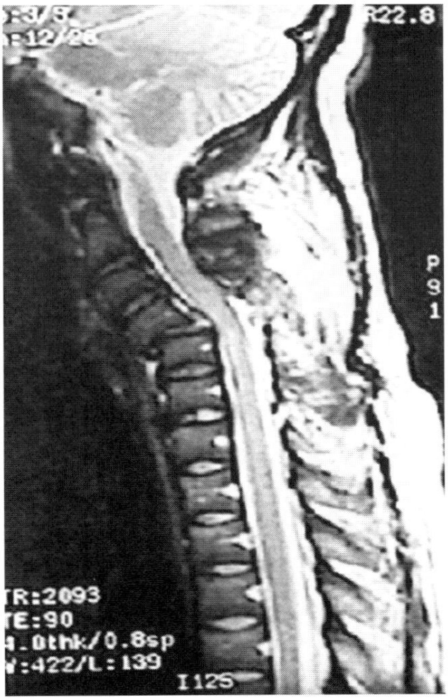

Figure 12–10 Flexion dislocation. Sagittal T2-weighted magnetic resonance imaging demonstrates the C4–5 subluxation and angulation. (With permission from Citow JS. Neuropathology and Neuroradiology: A Review. *New York, NY: Thieme Medical Publishers; 2001:214, Fig. 303.)*

XXI. Cervical Orthotics

A. Philadelphia collar—most effective for decreasing motion in the lower cervical spine (C5–T1)

B. SOMI brace—most effective for reducing flexion in the upper cervical spine

C. Minerva brace—most effective for midcervical instability

D. Halo vest—most effective for instability at C1–2 or C5–T1, but allows a swan-neck deformity at the midcervical spine (C3–5)

XXII. Thoracolumbar Fractures

A. Denis three-column model

1. Anterior column—ALL and $\frac{1}{2}$ disk
2. Middle column—PLL and $\frac{1}{2}$ disk
3. Posterior column—facets, laminas, spinous processes, and associated ligaments

B. Two-column injury considered unstable

C. Compression fracture

1. Only anterior column is injured
2. Considered unstable if vertebral height is decreased > 50% or there is > 30 degrees angulation
3. Treatment—brace (TLSO) or surgical stabilization (anterior or posterior approach)

D. Burst fracture

1. Both the anterior and middle columns are injured.
2. Considered unstable if vertebral height is decreased < 50%, the angulation is > 20 degrees, or there is > 50% canal compromise
3. Treatment—TLSO brace (3–6 months) or surgical decompression and stabilization (anterior approach is preferred over a posterior approach)
4. L5 burst fracture is difficult to instrument anteriorly; consider L4–S1 posterior fusion and TLSO brace with thigh cuff in 10 degrees flexion (Fig. 12–11A,B)

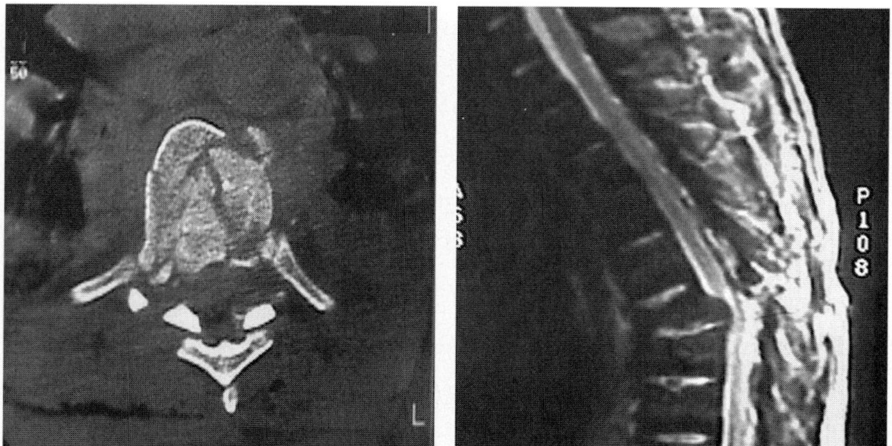

Figure 12–11 Burst fracture. (A) Axial computed tomography and (B) sagittal T2-weighted magnetic resonance imaging demonstrate angulation with retropulsion at T9. (With permission from Citow JS. Neuropathology and Neuroradiology: A Review. *New York, NY: Thieme Medical Publishers; 2001:215, Fig. 305.)*

E. Seat-belt fracture

1. Both the middle and posterior columns are injured.
2. Evaluation—sagittal CT reconstructions
3. Treatment—posterior instrumented fusion
4. Chance fracture—through vertebral bodies.

F. Fracture-dislocation—three-column injury requiring anterior and posterior stabilization

G. Instrumentation

1. Pedicle screws may be placed from C7 through the sacrum.
2. Exposure—must extend to tip of transverse processes to allow decortication of transverse processes and lateral facets
3. Entrance site—junction of medial transverse process and superior articulating process.
4. Awl is used to open into the pedicle
5. Fluoroscopy is used to place screws (5.5 or 6.5 mm) parallel to end plates and ending 80% into vertebral body
6. Intraoperative monitoring is used to stimulate screws to make sure there is no violation of cortex with pressure on a nerve root
7. Rod–hook systems may also be used in the thoracic and lumbar spines with pedicle hooks (up only), transverse process hooks (down only), or laminar hooks (up or down).
8. Rod–hook systems may be connected to pedicle screws.
9. Instrumentation should extend three levels above and two levels below the injury.
10. Construct may need to be extended to avoid ending at a transition level (cervicothoracic, thoracolumbar, or lumbosacral) or at a thoracic kyphosis.
11. Space lateral to facets should be packed with morselized bone
12. Anterior instrumentation with plates or rods involves bicortical screws (Fig. 12–12A,B).

H. Approaches

1. Upper thoracic spine—transsternal

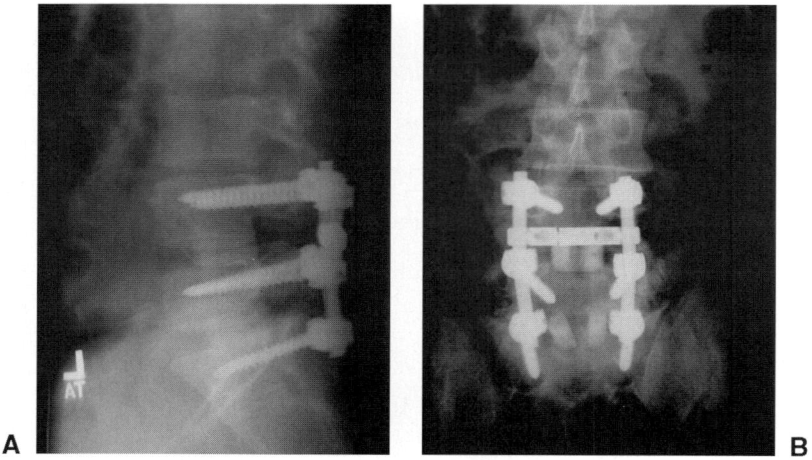

Figure 12–12 (A) Lateral x-ray of L4–S1 pedicle screw fusion with Tangent bony posterior lumbar interbody fusion (PLIF). (B) Anteroposterior x-ray of L4–S1 pedicle screw fusion with Tangent bony PLIFs.

2. Midthoracic spine T4–6—right transthoracic to avoid heart, use double lumen ET tube to deflate one lung
3. Lower thoracic spine to L2—left transthoracic, incise two levels above fracture site
4. Lumbar spine—left retroperitoneal to avoid liver and vena cava
   a. Retroperitoneal approach—lateral position
      i. Divide left anterior abdominal muscles down to preperitoneal fat and dissect laterally cutting latissimus dorsi to expose quadratus lumborum and iliopsoas medially
      ii. Sweep sympathetic chain laterally and ureter medially
      iii. Clip aortic radicular arteries as needed
      iv. Remove fractured bone and adjacent disks leaving contralateral cortex intact
      v. Distract intervertebral space with pins
      vi. Place a cage filled with bone graft, and secure with anterolateral plates (i.e., Kaneda) (Figs. 12–13, 12–14).
5. Lateral extracavitary, costotransversectomy, and transpedicular approaches can be used to decompress and possibly place an anterior cage or strut graft, but not instrumentation.

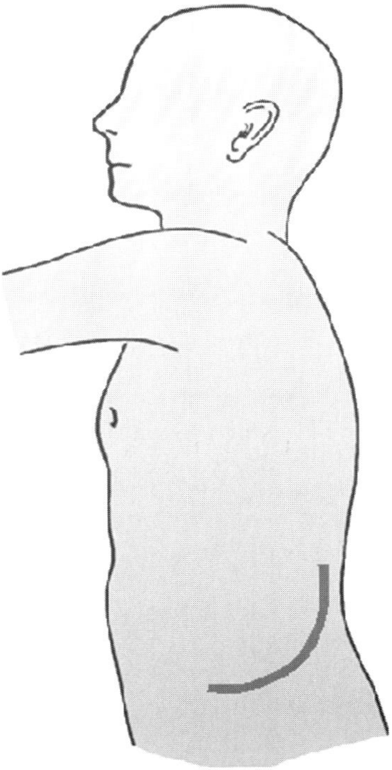

Figure 12–13 Retroperitoneal approach.

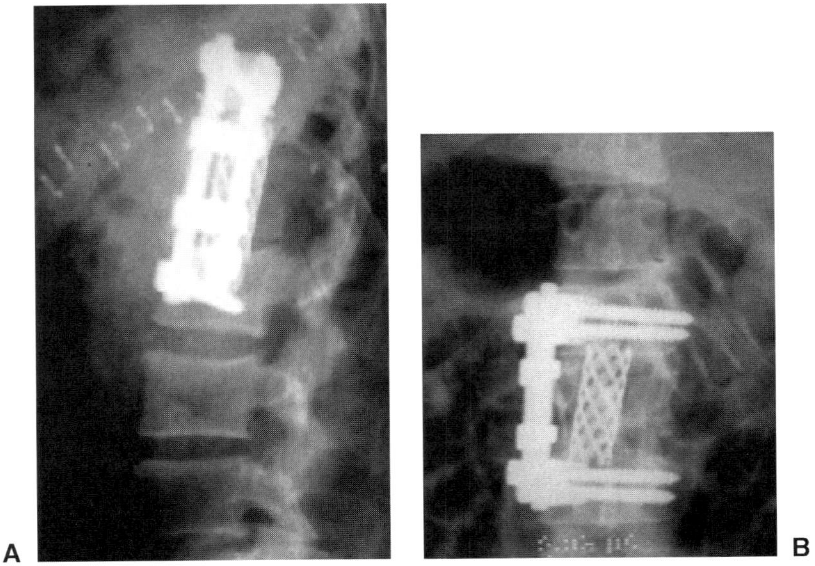

Figure 12–14 (A) Lateral x-ray of Kaneda plate fusion. (B) Anteroposterior x-ray of Kaneda plate fusion.

I. Pathological fractures

1. If mechanism not severe enough to explain the bony destruction, consider a tumor, infection, or osteoporosis
2. Evaluation—MRI, ESR, bone scan, and CXR

XXIII. Osteoporosis

A. Evaluation—bone mineral density and DEXA scan of proximal femur and lumbosacral spine.

1. Rule out hyperthyroidism, increased PTH, steroids, and tumor.

B. Treatment

1. Exercise
2. Calcium
3. Estrogen
    a. Increases DVT risk, possibly increases breast cancer risk, and decreases coronary artery disease
    b. Add progesterone to decrease endometrial carcinoma risk
4. Vitamin D
5. Calcitonin
6. Fosamax—decreases bone resorption

C. Compression fractures

1. Treatment
    a. Bracing or vertebroplasty—methylmethacrylate injected to decrease pain; also used for pathological fractures and hemangiomas
    b. Surgery—rarely needed

XXIV. Gunshot Wounds

A. Treatment

1. Surgery—useful only for incomplete spinal cord injury, CSF leak, instability (rare), or copper bullets

2. Colon perforation with CSF leak—explore to clean and pack the defect (80% infection rate)
3. Gastric and small bowel injuries are less contaminated.
    a. Use antibiotics but not steroids.
4. Lead from the bullet may rarely cause lead poisoning with neuropathy, encephalopathy, anemia, abdominal pain, and renal dysfunction.

CHAPTER 13

SPINAL DEGENERATIVE DISEASE

I. EVALUATION

A. Motor exam—deltoid (C5), biceps (C5,6), triceps (C7,8), wrist extension (C6), finger extension (C7), finger flexion (C8), interosseous (T1), hip flexion (L2), knee extension (L4), dorsiflexion (L4), extensor hallucis longus (L5), and plantar flexion (S1). (Also see section on footdrop.)

B. Sensory exam (Fig. 13–1)

1. Key levels—C1 (no sensory branch), C2 (posterior head), C6 (thumb), C8 (pinky), T4 (nipples), T10 (umbilicus), L4 (anterior knee), L5 (big toe), and S1 (lateral foot)

C. Deep tendon reflexes—biceps (C5,6), triceps (C7,8), brachioradialis (C6), patellar (L4), and Achilles' (S1)

II. CERVICAL DISK DISEASE

A. Signs/Symptoms

1. Radiculopathy—neck and interscapular pain, radicular arm pain, numbness and paresthesias, and lower motor neuron weakness

2. Myelopathy—upper motor neuron weakness, a sensory level, and incontinence. C8 and T1 radiculopathies may cause a partial Horner's syndrome.

B. Evaluation

1. MRI

2. Nerve conduction study—occasionally useful to differentiate radiculopathy from neuropathy.

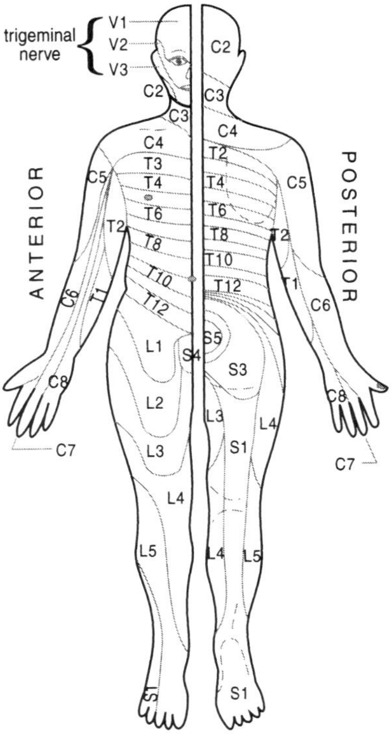

Figure 13–1 *Dermatome chart. (With permission from Greenberg MS.* Handbook of Neurosurgery. *5th ed. New York, NY: Thieme Medical Publishers; 2001:974.)*

3. Lhermitte's sign—neck flexion causes caudal electrical shocks; often seen with multiple sclerosis and SCSD
4. Spurling's sign—pressing the vertex of the head with the head extended and tilted to the symptomatic side reproduces radicular pain

C. Treatment

1. 90% of patients with acute cervical radiculopathy improve by 6 weeks with nonspecific conservative management.
2. Useful medical therapy—oral steroids (Medrol dose pack), NSAIDs, antispasmodics (for neck spasm), narcotics
3. Steroid side effects—avascular necrosis, mood changes, hypertension, glucose intolerance
4. Physical therapy for range of motion and traction exercises may be helpful.
5. Epidural steroids—not of clear benefit

6. Anterior cervical diskectomy and fusion—consider for patients who have significant weakness, long tract signs (bladder dysfunction), or debilitating pain, or who have failed conservative management
7. Posterior keyhole laminotomy with partial diskectomy for soft lateral disks—avoids the need for a fusion (consider with professional singers)
8. Plating—probably useful for two- and three-level procedures, though not proven for one-level fusions (Fig. 13–2)
9. Hard cervical collar—usually used post-op for 6 weeks

D. Complications

1. Anterior procedure may cause injury to the esophagus, trachea, recurrent laryngeal nerve (hoarseness or vocal cord paresis), or the carotid or vertebral artery (treat with direct repair or balloon trapping).
2. CSF leak—treat with fibrin glue and lumbar drain
3. Horner's syndrome—by dissection lateral to the longus coli

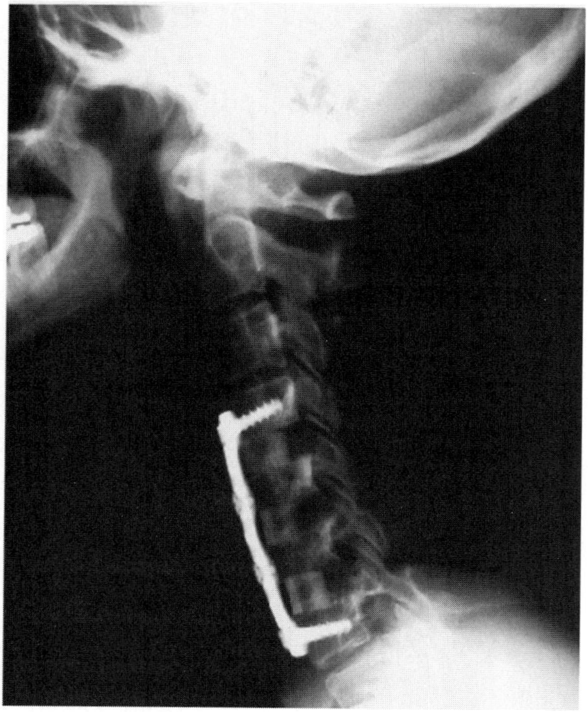

Figure 13–2 Lateral x-ray of C4–5, 5–6, and 6–7 cervical diskectomy and fusion.

4. Spinal cord injury—avoid by limiting extension with intubation; use fiberoptic technique
5. Sleep apnea or bradycardia (rare) with C3–4 level procedures

III. Cervical Spondylytic Myelopathy

A. Signs/Symptoms—as above but more often myelopathy (usually when the canal is <12 mm and rarely when it is >16 mm).
   1. Caused by direct neural compression, ischemia, and microtrauma.
   2. There may be a central cord syndrome.

B. Evaluation
   1. MRI and CT (better bony detail)
   2. Myelography—may be helpful, use Omnipaque 180 (lumbar) or 300 (cervical)
      a. Avoid these medications if the patient is taking Metformin (also stop it 3 days pre-op).
   3. Rule out—ALS (no sensory deficit, tongue fasciculations, distal fasciculations, or neck pain), multiple sclerosis, and subacute combined systems disease

C. Treatment
   1. Usually—anterior cervical diskectomy and removal of osteophytes around canal and foramen
   2. Less often—full corpectomies
   3. Consider posterior decompression if more than three levels are symptomatic or the pathology is mainly posterior.
   4. Avoid posterior procedures if there is no lordotic curvature.
   5. Posterior decompression—precipitates swan-neck deformity in 30% of cases (try to avoid by leaving the soft tissue on the facets) and does not stop progression of osteophytes.
   6. If both anterior and posterior approaches are needed, perform the anterior decompression and fusion first and follow with the posterior procedure in 8 weeks (consider supplemental fusion with lateral mass plates).

7. Anterior corpectomy complications—C5 radiculopathy (by posterior migration of the spinal cord or root traction) and worsened myelopathy 5%
8. If there is a nonunion after an anterior procedure, fix with a posterior tension band fusion (lateral mass plates or interspinous wiring).
9. Success rate of surgery—improved 60%, unchanged 25%, worse 15%

D. Ossified posterior longitudinal ligament

1. Treatment
    a. Decompress with anterior corpectomy followed by fusion.
    b. Postsurgery—use a collar for 3 months.
    c. Complication rate includes increased deficit 10%, failure to fuse 10%, and dural tear 25%.
    d. CSF leaks—common and should be treated with fibrin glue and lumbar drainage (usually temporary) (Fig. 13–3A,B)

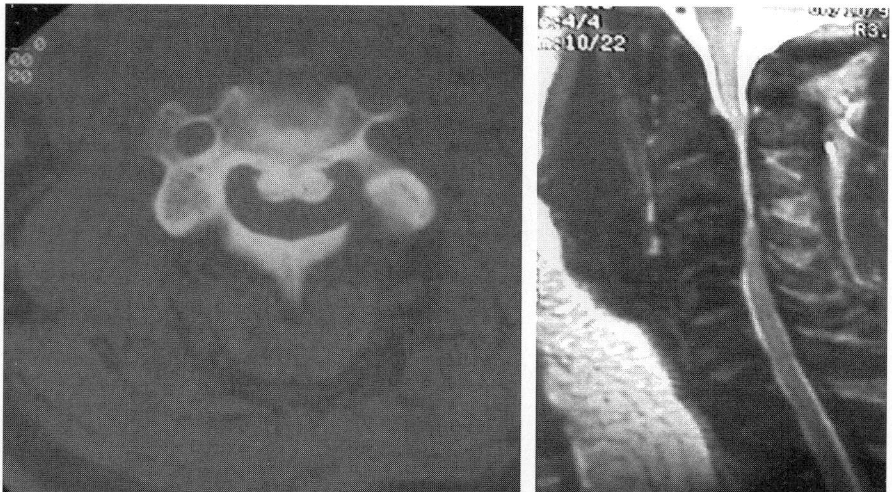

Figure 13–3 Ossified posterior longitudinal ligament (OPLL). (A) Axial computed tomgraphic bone window and (B) sagittal T2-weighted magnetic resonance imaging demonstrate C2–5 PLL calcification with cord compression. (With permission from Citow JS. Neuropathology and Neuroradiology: A Review. *New York, NY: Thieme Medical Publishers; 2001:208, Fig. 292.)*

IV. Upper Cervical Spine Diseases

A. Ankylosing spondylitis

1. Most often occurs in young males
2. Associated with rheumatoid arthritis and HLA-B27
3. Many spinal levels may fuse, but it spares the occipitoatlas and atlantoaxial joints.
4. Joints may be unstable
5. Frequent cause of lower back pain with sacroiliac erosion

B. Down syndrome—patients often develop atlantoaxial dislocation and cervical stenosis.

C. Morquio's syndrome—patients often develop atlantoaxial subluxation by hypoplasia of the dens and ligamentous laxity.

D. Rheumatoid arthritis

1. 80% of patients have cervical spine involvement.
2. Causes synovial proliferation with destruction of bone and ligaments
3. Atlantoaxial subluxation—occurs in 25% of patients
   a. Transverse ligament attachment becomes loose and symptoms are produced by a compressive pannus and instability.
   b. Atlantodental interval (ADI) should be < 4 mm if the transverse ligament is not lax.
   c. Treatment—C1–2 fusion if ADI > 6 mm or patient is symptomatic (a Brook's fusion with sublaminar wires and possible transarticular screws to add stability)
   d. Dislocation may need to be reduced before surgery with up to 7 days of traction with 5–15 lbs.
   e. Occiput–C2 fusion may be needed if C1 laminectomy is required for decompression or if the injury is unstable (there are frequent C1 arch fractures).
   f. May be necessary to perform a dens resection before or after stabilization.
   g. Failure of fusion—up to 50% of cases

h. Use a halo until the level is fused, around 12 weeks.

   i. Before removing the halo ring, check a flexion–extension x-ray.

i. Operative mortality—15%, mainly due to cardiac and pulmonary issues

4. Basilar impression

   a. Degenerative condition with ventral compression of the spinal cord or lower brain stem by skull settling over the dens

   b. Signs/Symptoms—headache and cranial nerve dysfunction

   c. Treatment—reduction with 7–15 lbs followed by transoral odontoidectomy and then occiput–C2 fusion

   d. If reducible—usually no need for anterior decompression

   e. Basilar invagination—congenital condition with a fusion of C1 to the occiput

      i. Not reducible with traction, but occasionally requires decompression

   f. Treatment—transoral odontoidectomy

      i. Perfomed supine with head in neutral position

      ii. Place the Crockard retractor (Codman) to move tongue caudally, soft palate rostrally, and endotracheal tube laterally.

      iii. Clean mouth with Betadine.

      iv. Palpate anterior tubercle of C1, inject posterior pharyngeal wall with lidocaine and epinephrine, and make longitudinal incision from above arch to base of C2.

      v. Retract pharyngeal tissue as one layer after subperiosteal dissection with Bovie.

      vi. Remove anterior arch of C1 and dens with a drill and pituitary forceps

      vii. Underlying soft tissue pannus may be carefully dissected off dura, but be careful to avoid a dural tear!

      viii. Close incision in one layer

      ix. Most patients will require a fusion (Figs. 13–4, 13–5).

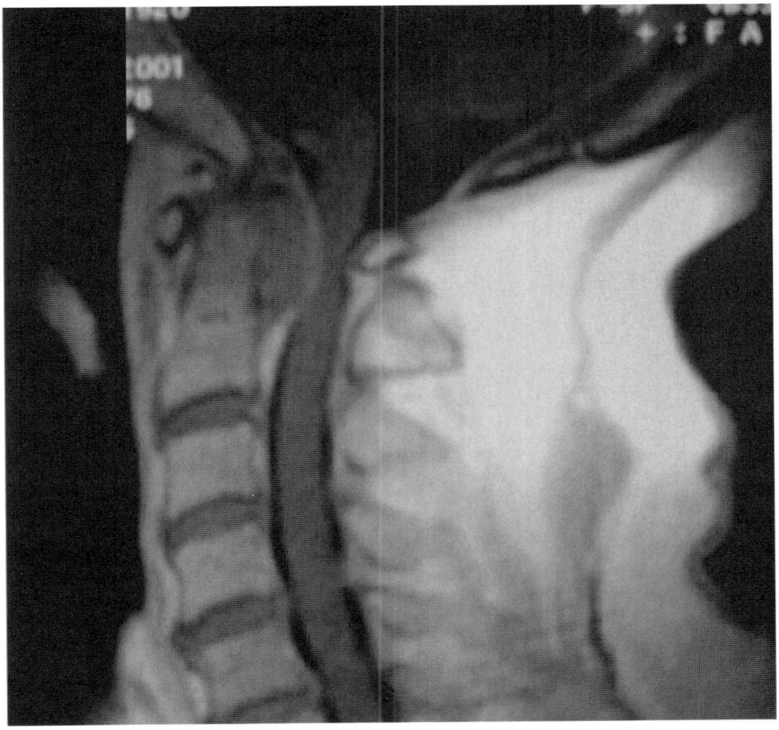

Figure 13–4 Sagittal T1-weighted magnetic resonance image with a large pannus posterior to the dens.

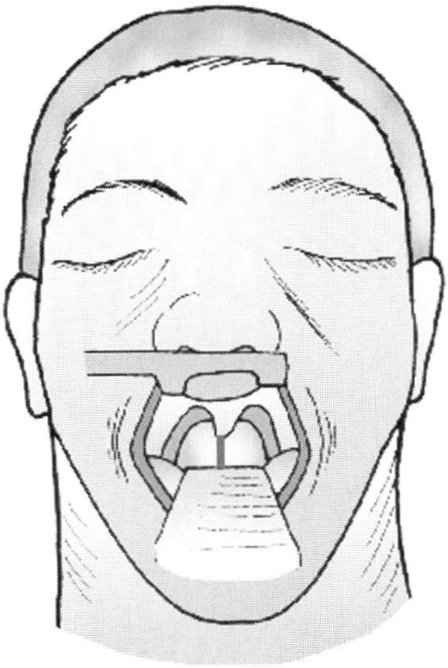

Figure 13–5 Transoral exposure and incision.

V. Thoracic Disk Disease

A. Posterolateral transpedicular approach—usually adequate exposure for most thoracic disks, but central disk removal is perfomed blindly with angled instruments (Woodson elevator)

1. Remove hemilamina above and below disk space as well as the facet joint.
2. Drill off pedicle from level below and clear out lateral and inferior disk space
3. Use Woodson elevator to push disk material down into the created trough

B. Costotransversectomy—allows direct line of vision to extend more medially

1. Initiate dissection as above; then remove transverse process and 4 cm of proximal adjacent rib
2. Complications—pneumothorax and radicular artery injury

C. Lateral extracavitary approach—allows better view of midline, but not as good as transthoracic approach

D. Transthoracic approach—best view for anterior pathology such as disk disease, burst fractures, or tumors

1. Upper T-spine—use transsternal approach
2. Middle T-spine—use right thoracotomy (avoid the heart)
3. Lower T-spine—use left thoracotomy
4. Thoracolumbar junction—use left retroperitoneal approach (avoid the liver)
5. Complications—radicular artery injury, pulmonary injury, and CSF-pleura fistula
6. Thoracoscopic approaches are gaining in popularity (Fig. 13–6).

VI. Lumbar Disk Disease

A. Signs/Symptoms—lower back and radicular leg pain, numbness, paresthesias, lower motor neuron weakness, and rarely incontinence.

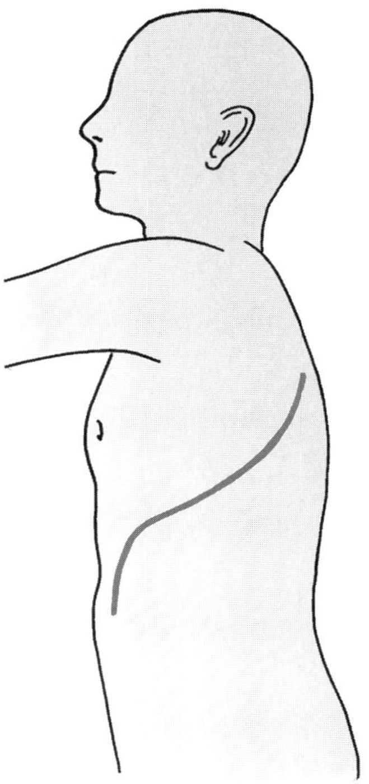

Figure 13–6 Transthoracic approach.

1. Cauda equina syndrome—saddle anesthesia and bladder and bowel incontinence or retention, usually due to a massive L5–S1 disk herniation

B. Evaluation

1. Straight leg raise (Lasègue's sign)—performed supine with leg straight to test lower lumbar roots (L5–S1)
2. Reverse straight leg raise—performed prone with flexed knees to test upper lumbar roots (L2–4)
3. MRI—most useful test
4. CT-myelography—reserved for more subtle pathology
5. NCV—needed (though rarely) to distinguish radiculopathy from neuropathy

C. Treatment

1. 90% of patients with acute lumbar radiculopathy improve by 6 weeks with nonspecific conservative management.
2. Useful medical therapy—same as for cervical disk disease
3. Physical therapy—to strengthen abdominal and back muscles will help prevent future back problems
4. Lumbar epidural steroid injections—may be helpful
5. Indications for early surgery—significant weakness, bowel or bladder dysfunction, or debilitating pain not controlled by narcotics
6. Gold standard procedure—microdiskectomy
7. For an extraforaminal (lateral) lumbar disk, there are two standard approaches.
    a. Hemilaminotomy to identify the nerve root followed by a complete facetectomy until the disk is identified
    b. Extrafacet approach with dissection over the lateral facets and transverse processes to find the nerve root and disk under the intertransverse ligament
    c. Iliac crest may need to be drilled down to reach the extruded disk

D. Complications

1. Infection 5%
2. Disk re-herniation 5%
3. Increased deficit 1–5%
4. Dural tear 10% (20% on reoperations)
5. Positioning pressure sore
6. Arachnoiditis—central adhesive nerve root cords or roots adherent to the dura seen on MRI
7. Deep vein thrombosis
8. Pulmonary embolism
9. Reflex sympathetic dystrophy 1%—occurs 4 days to 20 weeks after surgery and treated with PT, steroids, and sympathetic blocks

10. Vessel injury (rarely)—aorta and vena cava bifurcate into iliac vessels at L4
11. Superficial infection—treat with antibiotics
12. Deep infection—usually requires debridement with closure over a drain
    a. Evaluate the infection with CBC, ESR, cultures, and infused MRI.

VII. Lumbar Stenosis

A. Signs/Symptoms
1. Similar to lumbar disk disease symptoms but usually with a more insidious onset
2. Often neurogenic claudication with leg pain and weakness exacerbated by ambulation and relieved over minutes by sitting or lying down
    a. This may be confused with vascular claudication that improves immediately with rest and is evaluated with lower extremity arterial Doppler studies and an ankle/brachial blood pressure < 0.6.
3. Thigh pain—can be caused by trochanteric bursitis or hip arthritis, but the pain should not extend past the knee and there should be no sensory loss.
4. Lateral recess syndrome—compression of the nerve root adjacent to the pedicle by an enlarged superior facet process (< 4 mm of AP space)

B. Evaluation—MRI and CT-myelography if needed

C. Treatment
1. Conservative management as with disk disease, though most will eventually require laminectomy with medial facetectomies and foraminotomies.
2. Try to leave as much of the facet as possible because 1–5% of patients become unstable after lumbar decompression.
3. Vertically aligned facets—more likely to become unstable
4. Fusion—not needed if 50% of facet is left intact and disk is untouched
5. Lumbar fusion—best performed with pedicle screws augmenting a bony lateral fusion over decorticated transverse processes

6. Posterior lumbar interbody fusion (PLIF) cages—may be placed to augment a posterior fusion with a tall disk space, but have not been proven to be an effective stand-alone device (this is an area of controversy)
7. Open or laproscopic anterior lumbar interbody fusion (ALIF) cages also may be used in place of a PLIF.
8. Incision for ALIF placement is at the lateral edge of the rectus abdominus with a retroperitoneal dissection and great vessel mobilization.
9. Pedicle screws—usually 5.5 or 6.5 mm in diameter and 40–55 mm in length
   a. Should be aimed 20 degrees medial at L5, 30 degrees medial at S1, and sink 80% into the body (as guided by fluoroscopy or an image-guided system) (See the lumbar trauma section for more information.)
10. 80% of patients are improved with surgery.

D. Complications—same as lumbar disk disease complications
   1. 10–20% of postfusion patients develop adjacent stenosis over 10 years.

VIII. SPONDYLOLISTHESIS—subluxation, may have a pars defect.

A. Spondylolysis refers to the defect without subluxation.

B. Spondylolisthesis varieties
   1. Isthmic—little degenerative changes, possibly traumatic, usually at L5–S1
   2. Dysplastic
   3. Degenerative—90% at L4–5 and most others at L3–4
   4. Traumatic
   5. Pathological

C. Evaluation—same as lumbar stenosis with flexion–extension x-rays to rule out instability

D. Treatment—as with lumbar stenosis with the addition of pedicle screws (though some reports suggest fusion not needed because most cases of degenerative spondylolisthesis do not slip more after decompression) (Fig. 12–2A,B)

E. Symptomatic spondylolysis (back pain)

1. Evaluation—dynamic studies and local injections into the pars (to determine if this is indeed the pain source)

2. Treatment—consider repairing the pars directly with a screw (avoiding a fusion) or performing the traditional fusion (most common treatment).

IX. Facet-Mediated Back Pain—very controversial

A. Signs/Symptoms—pain is mainly in the paraspinal lower back without radicular pain.

B. Evaluation—MRI (rule out tumor or infection) and dynamic x-ray (rule out instability).

C. Treatment—physical therapy and NSAIDs

1. Refractory cases may be treated with radiofrequency facet denervation (controversial) or fusion.

X. Coccydynia

A. Signs/Symptoms—local tenderness over the coccyx

B. Evaluation—MRI and ESR

C. Treatment—NSAIDs, doughnut cushion, injections, and possibly resection (low success rates)

XI. Myelopathy Differential Diagnosis—see neurology section

A. Spinal cord compression—disk, bone, tumor, abscess

B. Spinal cord tumor

C. ALS—tongue fasciculations, normal sensation

D. Transverse myelitis

E. Spinal cord CVA—aortic dissection

F. Syphilis—tabes dorsalis

G. Subacute combined system disease

XII. Femoral Neuropathy—the femoral nerve arises from L2,3, and 4 to supply sensation to the anterior thigh and innervate the iliopsoas and quadriceps muscles.

A. Thigh adductors—not weak with a femoral neuropathy; they are innervated by the obturator nerve (L2,3)

B. L4 radiculopathy should have sensory loss from knee to medial malleolus (not anterior thigh), normal iliopsoas strength, and weakness of quadriceps, ankle dorsiflexion, and thigh adductors.

XIII. Footdrop—Usually from an L4 or 5 radiculopathy (painful) or a common peroneal nerve palsy (painless, normal gluteus medius strength with internal rotation of flexed hip and normal foot inversion); parasagittal meningioma may also present with footdrop

A. Superficial peroneal nerve (L4,5)—foot eversion and sensation to the dorsum of the foot

B. Deep peroneal nerve (L4,5)—dorsiflexion and a small area of sensation at the big toe web space

C. Tibial nerve (L5,S1)—foot inversion and plantar flexion with sensation to the sole of the foot

D. L5 proximal branches—gluteus medius (L4,5) for internal thigh rotation and gluteus maximus (L5–S1) to resist SLR

E. Sciatic nerve injury proximal to the peroneal division produces flail foot (no plantar- or dorsiflexion).

XIV. Syringomyelia

A. Communicating—central canal is patent (i.e., Chiari malformation)

B. Noncommunicating—trauma or tumor

C. Signs/Symptoms—capelike, suspended, dissociated sensory loss (of pain and temperature); pain; Charcot's joint; upper motor neuron findings in the lower extremities and lower motor neuron findings in the upper extremities

D. Evaluation—MRI and possibly cine-MRI

E. Treatment—occipitocervical decompression with duraplasty in the presence of a Chiari malformation (over 80% of theses syrinxes will resolve without shunting)

   1. Other types of syrinxes—treat by local decompression if possible or syringoperitoneal shunting (midline or dorsal root entry zone incision with 26-gauge tubing)

   2. Syringosubarachnoid shunting—less successful

XV. Paget's Disease

A. Cause—increased resorption of bone and replacement with irregular weak bone

B. Signs/Symptoms—bone pain, fractures, back pain, and deafness.

   1. Occurs in the skull, axial, and long bones

   2. Rarely develops into a sarcoma

C. Evaluation—increased serum alkaline phosphatase, normal calcium, increased urine hydroxyproline from cartilage, bone scan, and x-ray (thickened bones and lytic skull)

D. Treatment—calcitonin, bisphosphonates, and surgical decompression (there is frequently much blood loss)

XVI. Spinal Arteriovenous Malformations

A. Type I—dural artery to a spinal vein in a foramina

   1. Most frequent type (70%)

   2. Usually occurs in older men

   3. Causes progressive myelopathy

4. Foix-Alajouanine syndrome—subacute necrotizing myelitis due to venous hypertension

B. Type II—glomus AVM is intramedullary

C. Type III—juvenile AVM is intra- and extramedullary.

1. Carries a worse prognosis

D. Type IV—intradural perimedullary AVF

1. Occurs in younger patients

2. Frequently hemorrhages

E. Evaluation—MRI and angiography

1. Type I and IV AVMs—usually in adults and present with progressive weakness by venous hypertension

2. Type II and III AVMs—usually in children and present with hemorrhage

F. Treatment—endovascular embolization of feeding vessel or open coagulation and division of feeding vessels.

1. Type 1 AVMs—radicular artery can be divided or clipped on the foramen

CHAPTER 14

Peripheral Nerves

I. Anatomy

A. Dorsal scapular nerve—rhomboids and levator scapula

B. Long thoracic nerve—serratus anterior

C. Suprascapular nerve—supra and infraspinatous

D. Thoracodorsal nerve—latissimus dorsi

E. Phrenic nerve (C3–5)—diaphragm

F. Axillary nerve—to deltoid and teres minor

G. Musculocutaneous nerve—to coracobrachialis, biceps, and brachialis

H. Radial nerve—to triceps, brachioradialis, and extensor carpi radialis longus and brevis

   1. Posterior interosseous nerve—supplies the supinator, extensor carpi ulnaris, extensor digitorum, extensor digiti minimi, extensor pollicis longus and brevis, extensor indicis, and abductor pollicis longus (not median nerve)

I. Median nerve—pronator teres, flexor carpi radialis, palmaris longus, flexor digitorum superficialis, abductor pollicis brevis, flexor pollicis brevis (also by ulnar nerve), opponens pollicis, and lumbricales 1 and 2

   1. Anterior interosseous nerve—supplies the flexor digitorum profundus 1 and 2, flexor pollicis longus, and pronator quadratus

J. Ulnar nerve—flexor carpi ulnaris, flexor digitorum profundus 3 and 4, abductor digiti minimi, opponens digiti minimi, flexor digiti minimi, lumbricales 3 and 4, dorsal and palmar interosseous, flexor pollicis brevis (also by the median nerve), and adductor pollicis

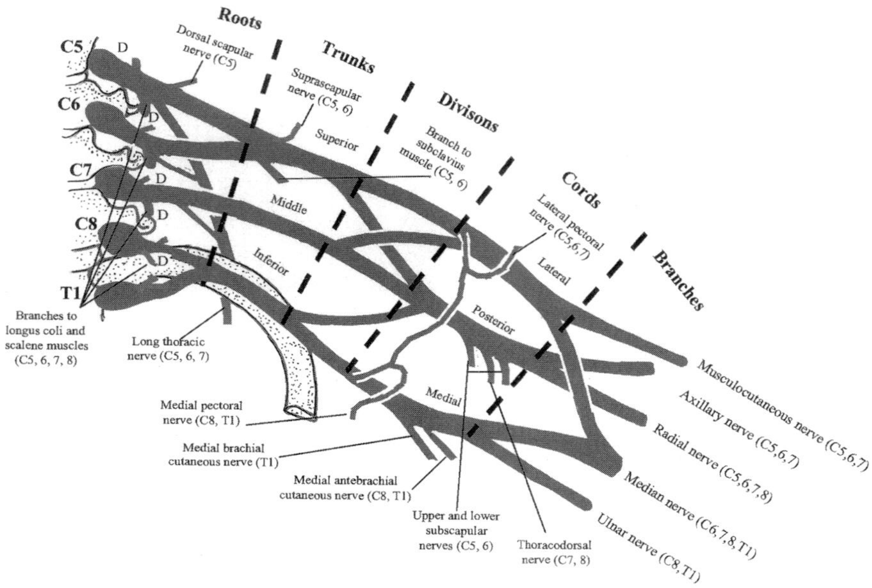

Figure 14–1 Brachial plexus anatomy. (With permission from Citow JS. Comprehensive Neurosurgical Board Review. *New York, NY: Thieme Medical Publishers; 2000:80, Fig. 1–44.)*

K. Brachial plexus (Fig. 14–1)

L. Superior gluteal nerve (L4–S1)—gluteus medius and minimus and tensor fascia lata

M. Inferior gluteal nerve (L5–S2)—gluteus maximus

N. Femoral nerve (L2–4)—iliacus, psoas, quadriceps femoris (rectus femoris and vastus lateralis, intermedius, and medialis), and sartorius

   1. There is also sensory innervation to the knee (anterior femoral cutaneous nerve) and medial knee to foot (saphenous nerve).

O. Obturator nerve (L2–4)—adductor brevis, adductor longus, adductor magnus (also by sciatic nerve), gracilis, and obturator externus

P. Sciatic nerve (L4–S3)—exits through the greater sciatic foramen to innervate the semimembranosus, semitendinosus, biceps femoris, and adductor magnus (also by the obturator nerve)

   1. Tibial nerve—gastrocnemius, soleus, tibialis posterior, flexor hallucis longus, and flexor digitorum longus

a. Medial plantar nerve—abductor hallucis, flexor digitorum brevis, and flexor hallucis brevis

b. Lateral plantar nerve—abductor digiti minimi, flexor digiti minimi, adductor hallucis, and interosseus muscles

2. Common peroneal nerve

a. Superficial peroneal nerve—peroneus longus and brevis

b. Deep peroneal nerve—tibialis anterior, extensor digitorum longus, extensor hallucis longus, peroneus tertius, and extensor digitorum brevis

3. Sensory branches—posterior femoral cutaneous nerve, tibial nerve (most of lower leg and sole of foot), and sural nerve (a small patch of lateral foot)

Q. Lateral femoral cutaneous nerve (L2,3)—sensation to lateral thigh

R. Pudendal nerve (S2–4)—sensation to perineum and external genitalia and motor to the external anal and urethral sphincters

S. Pelvic nerves (S2–4)—parasympathetic input for bowel, bladder, and sexual function

T. Miscellaneous sensory nerves—subcostal (T12), iliohypogastric (L1), ilioinguinal (L1), and genitofemoral (L1,2)

II. Entrapment Syndromes

A. Greater occipital neuralgia—from a C2 sensory branch

1. Superior nuchal trigger point—2.5 cm lateral and below the external occipital protuberance near the occipital artery

2. C1 or C2 fracture or subluxation—may crush the dorsal root ganglia

3. Treatment—usually with a nerve block using local anesthesia and steroids (10 mL 1% Marcaine and 40 mg Depo-Medrol)

1. Surgery—can be performed to avulse the nerve beyond the transverse process of C2 and the inferior oblique muscle (rarely needed)

B. Carpal tunnel syndrome—median nerve entrapment at the wrist by the transverse carpal ligament

1. Anatomy
   a. Median nerve—passes between the two heads of the pronator teres in the upper forearm
   b. Anterior interosseus nerve branch—supplies motor innervation for wrist and finger flexion
   c. Median nerve—passes under transverse carpal ligament (TCL) medial to flexor carpi radialis tendon, lateral to palmaris longus tendon, and above tendons of flexor digitorum superficialis and profundus
   d. Recurrent motor branch—normally arises under TCL (though rarely it runs through it) to supply lumbricales 1 and 2, opponens pollicis, and abductor and flexor pollicis brevis (LOAF) muscles
   e. Palmar cutaneous branch—arises from radial side of nerve 5 cm proximal to TCL and passes above it
   f. TCL—extends from palm to 3 cm beyond distal wrist crease
2. Cause—most cases related to repetitive hand motion
   a. Acute severe carpal tunnel syndrome may be caused by thrombosis of a persistent median artery or a local hematoma.
   b. Associated conditions—acromegaly, amyloid, multiple myeloma, hypothyroidism, diabetes, mucopolysaccharidosis, rheumatoid arthritis, and pregnancy
3. Signs/Symptoms
   a. Dysesthesias (usually nocturnal) involving the palmar side of the thumb, index and middle fingers, and half of the ring finger
   b. Sensory loss
   c. Weakness of the LOAF muscles
   d. Thenar atrophy
   e. Characteristic splitting of sensation of the fourth finger does not occur with nerve root or plexus lesions.
4. Evaluation
   a. History
   b. Motor evaluation—especially opponens of thumb to middle finger and thumb elevation/abduction

c. Tinel's sign—tapping over TCL

d. Phalen's maneuver—symptoms reproduced by wrist flexion

e. NCV—prolonged distal latency > 3.7

f. Thyroid panel, growth hormone, CBC (for myeloma), glucose, and renal panel

g. Laboratory evaluation—usually reserved for young patients with no history of repetitive hand movements

5. Treatment

a. Most cases resolve with conservative management such as rest, NSAIDs, neutral position splinting, and steroid injections (in line with the ring finger medial to the palmaris longus tendon to avoid injuring the nerve).

b. Surgery—involves division of the TCL

i. Incision—from distal wrist crease to base of thumb in line with web space between third and fourth digits

ii. Care is taken to avoid sectioning the palmar cutaneous branch on the radial side of the nerve.

iii. To section entire TCL—scissors should be used to undercut 3 cm proximal to wrist crease and distally into hand until there is loss of resistance

iv. Endoscopic division of TCL—also an option (Fig. 14–2)

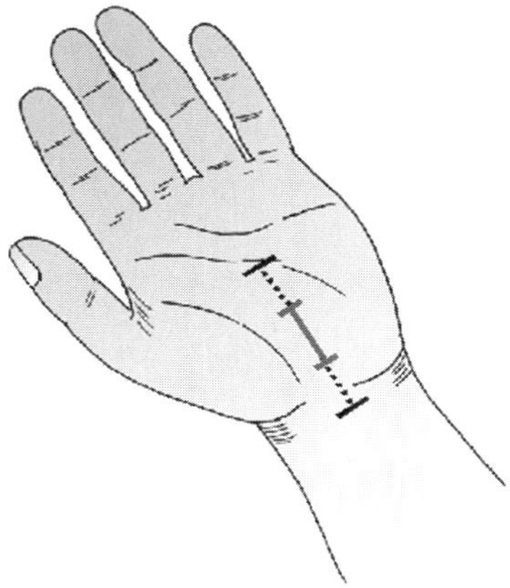

Figure 14–2 Carpal tunnel incision.

6. Complications
   a. Section of palmar cutaneous branch or motor branch
   b. Damage to median nerve
   c. Delayed neuroma or hypertrophic scar formation
   d. Insufficient release of TCL
   e. Reflex sympathetic dystrophy—rare, usually self-limited in 2 weeks, and treated with phentolamine IV or a sympathetic block

C. Pronator teres syndrome—entrapment of median nerve in forearm between the two heads of the pronator teres. The median nerve may also rarely be compressed in the upper arm at Struthers' ligament connecting the medial epicondyle and the supracondylar process (an anatomic variant located 5–7 cm proximal to the medial epicondyle).
   1. Causes—repetitive pronation or direct trauma
   2. Signs/Symptoms—aching and fatiguing with grip weakness and median distribution paresthesias
      a. No characteristic nocturnal exacerbations
      b. Numbness in the palm; not seen with carpal tunnel syndrome because the palmar cutaneous branch travels over the TCL
   3. Treatment—conservative, with surgery reserved for rare progressive cases.

D. Anterior interosseous syndrome—dysfunction of the anterior interosseous nerve, a branch of the median nerve innervating the flexor digitorum profundus 1 and 2, flexor pollicis longus, and pronator quadratus
   1. "Pinch sign" may be seen with poor flexion of the thumb and distal phalanges
   2. No sensory loss
   3. Most cases resolve in 8–12 weeks with conservative management.

E. Ulnar nerve entrapment—usually occurs at the elbow
   1. Signs/Symptoms—hand weakness, hypothenar and interosseus wasting, claw deformity (by weakness of lumbicales 3 and 4), and sensory loss and paresthesias of the medial hand, pinky, and medial half of the ring finger (Fig. 14–3)

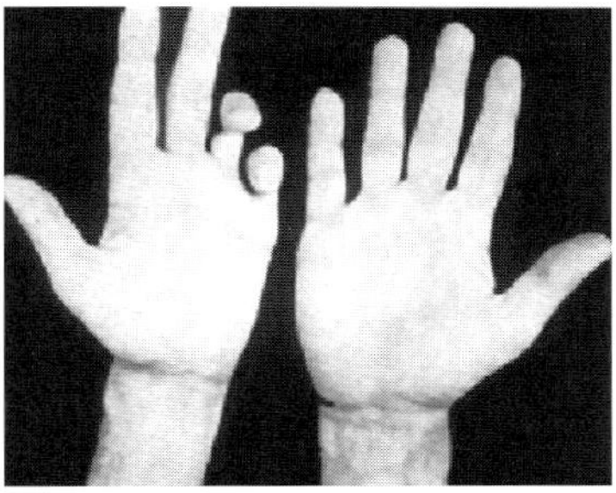

Figure 14–3 Claw hand photo.

2. Evaluation—Tinel's sign at the elbow, examination of finger abduction and digits 4 and 5 flexion, sensory examination (two-point discrimination is the most sensitive), and NCV
3. Treatment
    a. Neurolysis with or without transposition—subcutaneous, intramuscular, or submuscular
    b. Medial condylectomy—seldom performed at this time
    c. Results appear similar with neurolysis alone and with submuscular transposition—excellent 60%, fair 25%, poor 15% (no improvement or continued worsening)
    d. Technique for submuscular transpostion
        i. Lazy incision ventral to medial epicondyle
        ii. Decompression of nerve across elbow
        iii. Opening cubital tunnel between the two heads of the flexor carpi ulnaris distally
        iv. Opening the arcade of Struthers' proximally (a flat band of aponeurotic tissue anterior to the medial head of the triceps)
        v. Flexor tendons mass is then divided and the nerve tucked underneath along the bone
        vi. Tendon mass is then repaired in a relaxed fashion to avoid compression of the nerve
        vii. Care should be taken to avoid sectioning articular branches and branches to the flexor carpi ulnaris (Fig. 14–4).

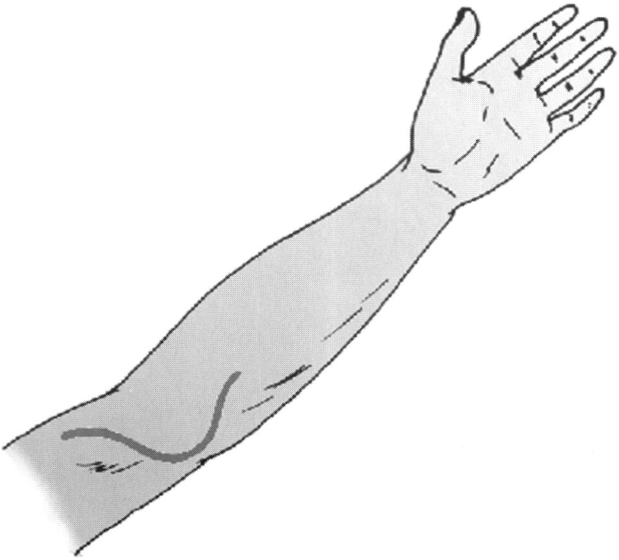

Figure 14–4 Ulnar nerve incision.

4. Entrapment at the wrist—in Guyon's canal above the transverse carpal ligament
   a. Rare and may be due to compression by a ganglion cyst
   b. No sensory loss in the dorsal hand and fingers because these nerve branches do not pass through the canal
5. Differentiate from C8 radiculopathy
   a. Radiculopathy is associated with neck pain, referred medial scapular pain, and more proximal arm pain.
   b. All of the intrinsic hand muscles should be weak, including the median nerve–innervated muscles.
   c. No sensory loss splitting the ring finger

F. Radial nerve entrapment—usually in the mid–upper arm (Saturday night palsy)
   1. Cause—operative positioning or a humerus fracture
   2. Signs/Symptoms—wristdrop without triceps weakness

a. Rule out lead poisoning.

b. Entrapment in the forearm at the arcade of Frohse may cause a posterior interosseous syndrome with finger extension weakness but no wristdrop or sensory loss.

c. Radial tunnel syndrome is due to compression in the supinator tunnel above and below the elbow and causes elbow pain with little muscle weakness. It may respond to decompression.

3. Evaluation—NCV; exploration indicated if there is no improvement in 8 weeks.

G. Suprascapular nerve entrapment—occurs in the suprascapular notch under the transverse scapular ligament

1. Signs/Symptoms—deep shoulder pain and supraspinatous and infraspinatous muscle atrophy

2. Treatment—surgical decompression is effective if conservative management fails.

H. Meralgia paresthetica (lateral femoral cutaneous nerve syndrome)

1. Cause—nerve entrapment under lateral inguinal ligament near anterosuperior iliac spine

a. Usually seen with obesity, diabetes, and pregnancy, and after surgery

2. Signs/Symptoms—burning dysesthesias over the lateral upper thigh

3. Evaluation—MRI and EMG

4. Treatment—weight loss, NSAIDs, steroid injections, or open section of the inguinal ligament

I. Peroneal nerve entrapment—usually due to compression of the common peroneal nerve at the fibular head. Symptoms include weakness of foot dorsiflexion and extensor hallucis longus, and less often foot eversion. Sensory loss is less common and involves the lateral aspect of the lower half of the leg. Evaluation is with MRI (rule out lumbar radiculopathy) and NCV. Footdrop may rarely be caused by a parasagittal brain tumor. Treatment is with decompression of the common peroneal nerve posterior to the fibular head, under the peroneus longus and above the soleus (Fig. 14–5).

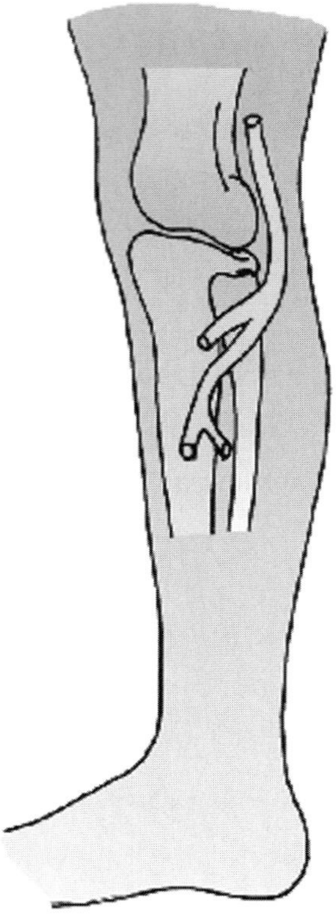

Figure 14–5 Peroneal nerve exposure.

J. Tarsal tunnel syndrome

1. Cause—posterior tibial nerve entrapment under medial malleolus
2. Signs/Symptoms—pain and paresthesias of the toes and sole of the foot and weakness of intrinsic foot muscles
3. Treatment—surgical decompression indicated if conservative management (i.e., ankle support) fails

III. Peripheral Neuropathy

A. Causes—DANG THE RAPIST—diabetes and drugs, amyloid, neoplasm and nutritional (B_{12}), Guillain-Barré syndrome, trauma, heredity, endocrine, electrolytes, and entrapment, renal and radiation, alcohol and AIDS, porphyria and paraneoplastic syndrome, infectious, immunologic, and ischemic, sarcoid, and toxins (i.e., lead)

B. Evaluation—glucose, Hb-a1c, TSH, ESR, B_{12}, NCV, EMG, and muscle and nerve biopsies

IV. Diabetic Neuropathy—may be sensory, motor, or autonomic

A. Most commonly involves the distal sensory nerves (stocking-glove sensory loss) or femoral nerve

B. Femoral neuropathy (which also may be caused by a psoas hematoma) is distinguished from an L4 radiculopathy by the presence of hip flexion weakness.

V. Charcot-Marie-Tooth Disease—inherited peroneal hypertrophic neuropathy causing peroneal-innervated muscle atrophy.

A. Onset—in adolesence

B. Distal muscle atrophy occurs first in the feet and then the hands (claw hand).

C. There is also sensory ataxia and weakness without autonomic dysfunction.

VI. Brachial Plexitis

A. Cause—autoimmune attack on the brachial plexus 2 weeks after an upper respiratory infection

1. May also be seen after radiation treatment or with diabetes

B. Signs/Symptoms—shoulder pain, numbness, paresthesias, and polyradicular weakness

C. Evaluation—NCV (demonstrates demyelination after 3 weeks) and a brachial plexus MRI and CXR (to rule out a structural lesion such as a Pancoast's or plexus tumor)

1. Pancoast's tumors usually involve the lower plexus.

D. Treatment—steroids; usually resolves over time

VII. Brachial Plexus Traumatic Injury

A. Preganglionic

1. Proximal to dorsal root ganglia
2. Not fixable

3. Associated with Horner's syndrome, serratus anterior paralysis with scapular winging, and rhomboid weakness from dorsal scapular injury

B. Postganglionic

1. May be amenable to nerve grafting procedures
2. Evaluation—EMG/NCV after 3 weeks
3. Erb-Duchenne palsy—C5–6 birth injury with proximal weakness and bellhop tip posture
4. Klumpke's palsy—C8–T1 injury from a fall or Pancoast's tumor causing a weak hand with claw deformity
5. T1 lesion may cause Horner's syndrome

VIII. Traumatic Neuropathy

A. Neuropraxia—functional loss without structural damage that lasts 6–8 weeks. Motor function usually affected more than sensation.

B. Axonotmesis—interruption of axons and myelin with intact perineurium and epineurium. Spontaneous regeneration may occur at 1–2 mm/d.

C. Neurotmesis—complete transection of the nerve and nerve sheath. Axonal regeneration may lead to neuroma formation.

D. Nerve repair

1. Perform immediately (to prevent retraction) only for a clean laceration with a very sharp object that will not crush the nerve (i.e., scalpel).
2. Otherwise, wait 3–6 weeks to explore to allow the scar to heal and the inflammation to resolve.
3. Evaluation—may include physical examination to determine the injured nerve, NCV, and MRI (to visualize continuity).
4. Treatment

    a. In surgery, perform nerve action potentials (NAP) over the neuroma to determine nerve continuity, and if positive, do only a neurolysis.

    b. Distal stump stimulation may be negative due to Wallerian degeneration, thus should not inhibit repair.

c. If NAP is negative, resect the neuroma until clean fascicles are seen and repair with nerve grafts (sural nerve, radial cutaneous nerve, intercostals nerve, etc.).

d. Earlier surgery preferred and if performed after 18 months, the muscle end plates may no longer be functional and the muscle may be fibrotic.

e. When cable grafting, shorter distances are more successful, and be sure to avoid tension.

f. Bioabsorbable polyglycol alcohol (PGA) tubes are now being used in place of nerve grafts.

g. Apply a splint if the repair crosses over a joint.

h. Results of repair will usually not be evident for 6 months.

i. For flail arm, consider an intercostal nerve to musculocutaneous nerve repair and a tendon transfer; arm fusion may be needed to prevent dislocation.

IX. Peripheral Nerve Tumors

A. Neuroma—not a neoplasm

1. Inflammatory mass consisting of tangled axons, Schwann cells, and fibroblasts

2. Usually painful and rubbery

B. Schwannoma

1. Firm, encapsulated, benign tumors growing eccentrically on the nerve with an epineurium capsule

2. Occur intracranially and along the spinal cord at the root entry zone of sensory nerves, in the head and neck, posterior mediastinum, retroperitoneum, and flexor surface of the extremities

3. Treatment—surgical resection when symptomatic

C. Neurofibroma

1. Fusiform, unencapsulated, benign tumors infiltrating the width of the nerve.

2. Cannot be completely removed without sacrificing the nerve

3. No reliable way to determine preoperatively whether the tumor is a schwannoma or a neurofibroma

D. Malignant peripheral nerve sheath tumor

1. Unlike benign tumors, usually painful and frequently cause motor deficit

2. 50% of patients have NF-1

3. Treatment—resection and radiation

E. Mass behind knee

1. Popliteal artery aneurysm

2. Ganglion (Baker's) cyst

3. Nerve sheath tumor—positive Tinel's sign, able to be moved side-to-side but not the length of the nerve, rarely with motor deficit unless malignant

CHAPTER 15

OPHTHALMOLOGY

I. Monocular Blindness—consider amaurosis fugax, optic neuritis, retinal detachment.

II. Optic Neuritis—usually seen with multiple sclerosis (especially if bilateral) and sarcoid.

A. Signs/Symptoms

1. Early stage—may appear as papilledema (blurred disk margins)
2. Later stage—may appear as optic atrophy (bright white optic disk with clean margins)

III. Diabetic 3rd Nerve Palsy (Vasculitic/Ischemic)—pupil sparing and painful

IV. Compressive 3rd Nerve Palsy—pupil dilated early and painless

V. Horner's Syndrome—ptosis, miosis, and anhydrosis

A. Sympathetic input to the head is through the superior cervical ganglion.

B. Spontaneous causes—arterial dissection and tumor

VI. Internuclear Ophthalmoplegia

A. Cause—medial longitudinal fasciculus dysfunction

B. Signs/Symptoms—contralateral medial rectus fails to move the eye medially to maintain conjugate gaze with the ipsilateral 6th nerve action (other 3rd nerve function is normal).

C. Frequently associated with MS (especially if bilateral) or CVA

VII. 6th Nerve Palsy

A. Causes—elevated ICP, diabetes, cavernous sinus lesion, or Dorello's canal inflammation

B. Gradenigo's syndrome—apical petrositis with 6th nerve palsy, V1-distribution retro-orbital pain, and a draining ear (due to infection)

VIII. Painful Ophthalmoplegia

A. Cause—often mucormycosis or diabetes

B. Tolosa-Hunt syndrome—granulomatous inflammation of the cavernous sinus and superior orbital fissure

IX. Painless Ophthalmoplegia—consider myasthenia grava.

X. Raeder's Paratrigeminal Neuralgia—partial Horner's syndrome (no anhydrosis) with numbness in the trigeminal distribution

XI. Syphilis—causes near-light dissociation; pupil accommodates but does not react

CHAPTER 16

Otology

I. Meniere's Disease (Endolymphatic Hydrops)

A. Signs/Symptoms—vertigo (5–30-minute episodes), emesis, tinnitus, and low-frequency hearing loss

B. Evaluation—electronystagmography, audiogram, and MRI.

C. Treatment—salt restriction, diuretics, Valium, Antivert, avoidance of caffeine, 8th nerve sectioning, and shunting of the endolymphatic sac

D. Rule out benign positional vertigo, vestibular schwannoma, and vestibular neuronitis.

II. Hearing Loss—use Rinne's test to differentiate conductive versus sensorineural hearing.

III. Tinnitus—consider glomus jugulare, dural AVF, and cavernous–carotid fistula.

IV. Facial Palsy

A. Causes—usually due to Bell's palsy, trauma, zoster, or tumor.

B. Treatment—repair with a direct anastomosis of XII, XI, or IX to VII.

V. Bell's Palsy

A. Cause—probably caused by a virus (usually HSV, occasionally by Lyme disease).

B. Treatment—steroids and eye protection (gold weight or tarsorrhaphy)

C. Spontaneous recovery occurs in 80% (10% only partial); improvement begins in 3 weeks.

VI. Branches of the Facial Nerve (From Proximal to Distal)—to geniculate ganglion (lacrimation), stapedial (hyperacusis), chorda tympani (salivation, taste), and facial motor.

VII. Decreased Facial Sensation—consider hypocalcemia.

CHAPTER 17

Helpful Hints

I. History should address infection or tumors.

II. New onset headaches should be evaluated with CT, LP (don't miss infection), and possibly angiogram.

III. Post-op leg pain should prompt search for DVT.

IV. Positional back pain may suggest instability.

V. Safe aneurysm surgery requires proximal control.

VI. All severe trauma patients should be immobilized with a cervical collar.

VII. Patients going to the operating room should have blood work (PT/PTT, CBC, electrolytes) and blood available.

VIII. Remember to mention medications used with surgery such as dexamethasone, Dilantin, mannitol, and antibiotics.

IX. Consider awake surgery with speech mapping for lesions involving the speech areas.

X. Consider nerve monitoring with vestibular schwannoma resection (cranial nerves V, VII, and VIII).

XI. For skull base surgical approaches, plan dural closure (i.e., periosteal flap).

XII. Be aggressive treating temporal hematomas, posterior fossa masses, and spinal cord compression.

XIII. Complications from most procedures involve damage to neural tissue (brain, spinal cord, roots, nerves) or vessels, CSF obstruction, and infection. Evaluate for blood clot, ischemia, infection, seizures, hyponatremia, and hydrocephalus.

XIV. Relax, there is little they will ask you that you have not treated successfully numerous times.

XV. This book is one person's view of things. It is not the gospel. Many competent neurosurgeons have differing views and there is no one correct answer. As long as the patients are well cared for, all will be fine.

Glossary

ABCs: airway, breathing, circulation

ABG: arterial blood gases

ACA: anterior cerebral artery

ACAS: asymptomatic carotid atherosclerosis study

ACh: acetylcholine

ACTH: adrenocorticotropic hormone

ADH: anti-diuretic hormone

ADI: atlantodental interval

AFB: acid-fast bacilli

AFib: atrial fibrillation

AFP: alpha fetal protein

AICA: anterior inferior cerebellar artery

AIDS: acquired immunodeficiency syndrome

ALIF: anterior lumbar interbody fusion

ALL: anterior longitudinal ligament

ALS: amyotrophic lateral sclerosis

AP: anteroposterior

ASA: aspirin

AVF: arteriovenous fistula

AVM: arteriovenous malformation

BAER: brain stem auditory evoked response

BBB: blood–brain barrier

BCNU: carmustine

BoTox: botulism toxin

BUN: blood urea nitrogen

CBC: complete blood count

CBF: cerebral blood flow

CCA: common carotid artery

CCF: carotid–cavernous fistula

CCNU: lomustine

CEA: carotid endarterectomy

CHF: congestive heart failure

CJD: Creutzfeldt-Jakob disease

$CMRO_2$: cerebral metabolic rate of oxygen

CNS: central nervous system

COPD: chronic obstructive pulmonary disease

COWS: cold opposite, warm same

CPK: creatine phosphokinase (2,3)

CPP: cerebral perfusion pressure

CRP: C-reactive protein

CSF: cerebrospinal fluid

CSW: cerebral salt wasting

CT: computed tomography

CVA: cerebrovascular accident

CVP: central venous pressure

CXR: chest x-ray

DANG THE RAPIST: diabetes and drugs; amyloid; neoplasm and nutritional (B_{12}); Guillain-Barré syndrome; trauma; hereditary; endocrine, electrolytes, and entrapment; renal and radiation; alcohol and AIDS; porphyria and paraneoplastic syndrome; infectious, immunologic, and ischemic; sarcoid; and toxins

DDAVP: desmopressin acetate

DI: diabetes insipidus

DIC: disseminated intravascular coagulopathy

DM: diabetes mellitus

DNA: deoxyribonucleic acid

DREZ: dorsal root entry zone

DVT: deep venous thrombosis

EAM: external acoustic meatus

EBV: Epstein-Barr virus

ECA: external carotid artery

EEG: electroencephalogram

EKG: electrocardiogram

ELISA: enzyme-linked immunosorbent assay

EMG: electromyogram

ENT: ear, nose, and throat

ER: emergency room

ESR: erythrocyte sedimentation rate

ET: endotracheal

ETOH: ethanol

FMD: fibromuscular dysplasia

FSH: follicle-stimulating hormone

GB: glioblastoma

GBM: glioblastoma multiforme

GCS: Glasgow coma scale

GH: growth hormone

GPi: globus pallidus interna (3,8)

GU: genitourinary

Gy: gray (unit of radiation)

HCT: hematocrit

HLA-B27: human leukocyte antigen-B27

HOB: head of bed

HSV: herpes simplex virus

HTN: hypertension

ICA: internal carotid artery

ICP: intracranial pressure (2,3)

Ig: immunoglobulin

IGF: insulin-like growth factor

INR: international normalized ratio

IQ: intelligence quotient

IVDA IV: drug abusers

JCV JC: virus

KUB: kidney, ureter, and bladder

LE: lower extremity

LH: luteinizing hormone

LINAC: linear accelerator

LOAF: lumbricales 1 and 2, opponens pollicis, and abductor and flexor pollicis brevis muscles

LP: lumbar puncture

MAO: monoamine oxidase

MCA: middle cerebral artery

MCV: mean corpuscular volume

MI: myocardial infarction

MM: myelomeningocele

MRA: magnetic resonance angiography

MRI: magnetic resonance imaging

MRV: magnetic resonance venography

MS: multiple sclerosis

NAP: nerve action potentials

NASCET: North American symptomatic carotid endarterectomy trial

NCV: nerve conduction velocity

NEJM: New England Journal of Medicine

NF: neurofibromatosis

NF-1: neurofibromatosis type 1

NG: nasogastric

NS: normal saline

NSAID: nonsteroidal anti-inflammatory drug

OCP: oral contraceptive pill

OFC: occipital-frontal circumference

OPLL: Ossified posterior longitudinal ligament

OR: operating room

PCA: posterior cerebral artery

PCOM: posterior communicating artery

PCR: polymerase chain reaction

PET: positron emission tomography

PGA: polyglycol alcohol

PICA: posterior inferior cerebellar artery

PLIF: posterior lumbar interbody fusion

PLL: posterior longitudinal ligament

PML: progressive multifocal leukoencephalopathy (3,5)

PMN: polymorphonuclear neutrophil

PNET: primitive neuroectodermal tumor

PNS: peripheral nervous system

PO: taken orally

PSNP: progressive supranuclear palsy

PT: prothrombin time

PT: physical therapy

PTH: parathyroid hormone

PTT: partial thromboplastin time

REZ: root entry zone

RIND: reversible ischemic neurological deficit

RPR: rapid plasma reagin

RSD: reflex sympathetic dystrophy

SACE: serum angiotensin-converting enzyme

SAH: subarachnoid hemorrhage

SATCHMO: sarcoid, aneurysm/adenoma (pituitary), teratoma, craniopharyngioma, hypothalamic hamartoma/histiocytosis X, meningioma, optic glioma

SBP: systolic blood pressure

SCD: sequential compression devices

SCIWORA: spinal cord injury without radiographic abnormality

SCM: sternocleidomastoid

SCSD: subacute combined systems disease

SG: specific gravity

SIADH: syndrome of inappropriate antidiuretic hormone (2,3)

SLE: systemic lupus erythematosis

SOMI: sternal-occipital-mandibular immobilizer

SPECT: single photon emission computed tomography

SQ: subcutaneous

SRS: stereotactic radiosurgery

SSEP: somatosensory evoked potential

SSPE: subacute sclerosing panencephalitis

STA: superficial temporal artery

TB: tuberculosis

TCL: transverse carpal ligament

TED: threshold erythema dose

TENS: transcutaneous electrical nerve stimulation

TIA: transient ischemic attack

TLSO: thoracolumbar spinal orthosis

t-PA: t-plasminogen activator

TSH: thyroid stimulating hormone

UE: upper extremity

UOP: urine output

VA: vertebral artery

V/Q: ventilation-perfusion

VDRL: Venereal Disease Research Laboratory

VIM: ventral intermediate thalamic nucleus

VIND: vascular, infectious, neoplastic, demyelinating

VMA: vanillylmandelic acid

VP: ventriculoperitoneal

WBCs: white blood cells

WBRT: whole brain radiation therapy

XRT: radiation therapy

Index